# BODY LOVE
# A JOURNAL

# BODY LOVE
## A JOURNAL

12 WEEKS
TO PRACTICE
POSITIVITY, CREATE
MOMENTUM,
AND BUILD YOUR
HEALTHY LIFESTYLE

## KELLY LeVEQUE

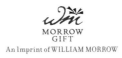

MORROW
GIFT
An Imprint of WILLIAM MORROW

This book contains advice and information relating to health care. It should be used to supplement rather than replace the advice of your doctor or another trained health professional. If you know or suspect you have a health problem, it is recommended that you seek your physician's advice before embarking on any medical program or treatment. All efforts have been made to assure the accuracy of the information contained in this book as of the date of publication. This publisher and the author disclaim liability for any medical outcomes that may occur as a result of applying the methods suggested in this book.

FIRST EDITION

Designed by Bonni Leon-Berman

Library of Congress Cataloging-in-Publication Data has been applied for.

ISBN 978-0-06-304898-0

20 21 22 23 24 RTLO 10 9 8 7 6 5 4 3 2

To my mom, my sisters, my best friends,

and all the women out there supporting

one another to live a nourished and

vibrant life. My hope is that this journal

helps you to practice compassion,

accomplish your goals, and follow a

purpose-driven path.

# CONTENTS

# INTRODUCTION

## CULTIVATING POSITIVITY

Welcome to your Body Love journal. Let me start by saying this journal is meant to be a holistic tool to help you positively track your food choices, cultivate gratitude, and clarify your goals in a way that deepens the love you have for yourself and your physical body. It is based on the principles found in my two books, *Body Love* and *Body Love Every Day*, as well as my work with private clients.

In the past, food journaling has been used to track calories and macros, promote restriction, and shame the journaler. In my practice, I have seen it strain my clients' relationships with food.

On the other hand, gratitude journaling, meal planning, and celebrating healthy food choices can create the opposite experience. Identifying novel and very specific things in your daily life you are grateful for increases your overall happiness levels and deepens your appreciation for simple joys, peaceful moments, and blessings. Being inspired by seasonal produce, motivated to learn a recipe, or enthusiastic about elevating a family favorite helps you continue to prioritize meals that nourish your mind, body, and soul. Research has even shown that feeling proud of your food choices releases dopamine in the brain and increases the chances you will repeat that behavior again and again. So it's time to start feeling good about our food choices!

This Body Love journal is meant to be a positive log of your life—the beautiful moments, the healthy choices, and the simple pleasures. It is here to help you embrace and celebrate meaningful moments without nitpicking—to remind you of your goals, solidify your nonnegotiables, and highlight your progress. The journal includes monthly, weekly, and daily tracking pages to help you clarify your goals, plan for progress, and celebrate your accomplishments.

*Monthly Manifestation* provides a place for self-reflection, forgiveness, and manifestation. The SMART goals exercise helps you put the dreams you have been manifesting into an actionable plan. As I mentioned in my first book, *Body Love,* we all have a few self-limiting beliefs and stories we tell ourselves. These can stand in the way of our true potential, dim our light, and cannibalize our ability to love ourselves, so please take the time to *go in* and *let go* during your monthly tracking—revisit these stories and rewrite them! If you didn't have these baked-in beliefs, where would you be? I know without a doubt you have unlimited potential for growth, you have the ability to build and live a healthy lifestyle, and your dreams are never too big. So, dream big—and then write down your SMART goals and go do that smart work!

*Weekly Planning* will motivate what's on your plate, inspire you to try new recipes, and keep you committed to the healthy activities that make you feel vibrant. Use the grocery list to help you stock your freezer, pantry, and fridge with all your favorite Fab Four foods; jot down the bulk proteins you plan to make for quick lunches; and double-check that you have everything you need to whip up your daily smoothies. A little prior planning ensures you will be prepared to make the healthy choice when you might feel tempted, overwhelmed, or stressed.

Last, weekly tracking asks you to start committing to anchor appointments. These are appointments you set with yourself that establish consistency in your week. A great example of an anchor appointment you might already keep would be a weekly religious service or therapy session. You go every week—it's almost automatic. Anchor appointments offer you the same cadence with your wellness. By committing to nonnegotiable weekly wellness appointments, you keep your commitment to the activities that enrich your life, nourish your body, and feed your soul, all without it ever feeling like work.

*Daily Expression* offers you food freedom, helps you organically weave gratitude into your daily practice, asks you to prioritize your hit list, and elevates your mood. The journal pages for daily tracking are designed to record the positive on your plate and in your life.

There are places to jot down what I call in my books and practice the Fab Four—the protein, fat, fiber, and greens—you've added to your plate, mark your water intake, and check off a wellness activity like meditation, yoga, or running. Please do not count calories, track macros, or shame your food choices; simply track the good stuff and celebrate the wins—and watch that create momentum. Did you add spinach to your smoothie? Jot it down! Did you save your celery tops and throw those in the blender too? Give yourself a high five! This type of tracking, with a laserlike focus on the positive, shifts your relationship with food, focuses on abundance instead of restriction, and helps you stay motivated to nourish yourself.

Positivity tracking is a type of gratitude journaling that requires you to be very specific about what you were most thankful for during your day. I highly suggest you cultivate this practice. The more you get used to looking for those moments, the more they appear in your life and the sweeter your days become. You'll begin to experience bath-time giggles, a quiet morning coffee, an acknowledgment at work, or a motivating mantra at your yoga class in a completely different way.

The hit list is short for a reason; these are the three highest-priority to-dos in your day. As women, we forget to put our own oxygen masks on first and we spread ourselves thin, overcommitting to engagements and supporting others without focusing on our own livelihoods as a priority. Every time you say yes to something when you feel like saying no, it's an indication that you are searching, looking for love and acceptance from an outside source instead of showing yourself respect. Ultimately, you'll be left feeling resentful if you aren't taking care of yourself. I'm here to tell you—you can be a loyal friend, supportive spouse, and caring parent while still prioritizing yourself and your goals. In fact, your actions are showing those around you how to respect themselves and their goals too. Remember, the hit list helps you hit your goals.

The *Parking Lot* is exactly what it sounds like: a wide-open space to park your thoughts, let go of anything holding you back, and release anxieties to clear your mind of debris. Like a traditional journal, this open space can be used to jot down a special memory or mantra, or simply be a place to manifest and dream daily.

This Body Love journal is a tangible tool to help you follow the light structure of the Fab Four, focus on the positive, and live with a grateful heart. It's my hope that this journal will enrich your life.

Be well,
*Kelly LeVeque*

# PART I

# RECIPES AND MORE

# FAB FOUR SMOOTHIES AND FAVORITES

To give you a taste of how easy and delicious it can be to add protein, fat, fiber, and greens to every meal, here is a curated list of Fab Four Smoothies and favorites my clients, readers, and family love!

Spa Day Fab Four Smoothie   13

Cookies and Cream Fab Four Smoothie   14

Original Green Fab Four Smoothie   15

Icy FAB-uccino   16

Stawberry Lemonade Smoothie   17

Herby Italian Chicken   18

Coconut Cauliflower Rice with Sweet Coconut
Chicken and Broccoli   20

Cowboy Skillet   22

Chicken Kale Cobb Snob Salad   23

Butter-Lettuce-Wrapped Shrimp Tacos   24

Roasted Black Bean Vegan Burgers   26

# Spa Day Fab Four Smoothie

Start the week fresh with this super-green #fab4smoothie. The lemon cuts any bitter taste from the spinach, and the mint and cucumber will make you feel like you just stepped into a spa.

Vanilla protein powder containing 20 to 30 grams protein
¼ to ½ cup diced avocado
1 to 2 tablespoons chia seeds
Juice of ½ to 1 lemon
A few fresh mint leaves
Handful of fresh spinach
1 small Persian cucumber
2 cups unsweetened nut milk

Place all the ingredients in a high-speed blender and blend, adding water as needed to reach your desired consistency.

# Cookies and Cream
# Fab Four Smoothie

This smoothie is proof that with a delicious protein powder and an appropriate serving size of fruit, you can have your dessert and eat it too! This is the perfect smoothie for when cravings hit.

Chocolate coconut Primal Kitchen Collagen Fuel powder
    containing 20 to 30 grams protein
1 tablespoon almond butter
1 tablespoon flaxseeds
Handful of fresh spinach
¼ cup frozen blueberries
1 to 2 cups unsweetened almond milk

Place all the ingredients in a high-speed blender and blend to your desired consistency.

# Original Green Fab Four Smoothie

A simple whole food smoothie that is balanced and filling nourishes your body and fuels you up for the day ahead.

Vanilla protein powder containing 20 to 30 grams protein
¼ avocado (or 2 tablespoons almond butter)
2 tablespoons chia seeds
Handful of fresh spinach
1 to 2 cups unsweetened nut milk

Place all the ingredients in a high-speed blender and blend to your desired consistency.

# Icy FAB-uccino

Attention, all coffee lovers! This smoothie is a balanced, antioxidant-rich, and icy treat sans guilt. Enjoy your coffee and your #fab4smoothie in one delicious icy cup.

Chocolate protein powder containing 20 to 30 grams protein

1 tablespoon almond butter

2 tablespoons chia seeds

1 tablespoon organic instant coffee grounds, or 1 packet Four Sigmatic Instant Mushroom Coffee with Lion's Mane

¼ cup frozen cauliflower rice

Handful of fresh spinach (optional)

1 to 2 cups unsweetened nut milk

Place all the ingredients in a high-speed blender and blend to your desired consistency.

# Strawberry Lemonade Smoothie

A fresh summer treat that will satisfy your nostalgic childhood cravings.

Vanilla protein powder containing 20 to 30 grams protein
1 tablespoon psyllium husk powder
¼ avocado
¼ cup strawberries
Juice of 1 lemon
Small handful fresh spinach
1 tablespoon lemon zest
1½ cups unsweetened nut milk or water

Place all the ingredients in a high-speed blender and blend to your desired consistency.

# Herby Italian Chicken

**MAKES 2 SERVINGS**

Tender, flavorful, and easy to cook, this Italian-style herbed chicken is perfectly paired with peppery arugula and juicy tomatoes, proving that simple techniques and fresh produce are all you need to feel satisfied.

2 (6- to 8-ounce) boneless, skinless organic chicken
   breasts, butterflied
2 garlic cloves, minced
2 teaspoons dried oregano
2 teaspoons dried thyme
2 tablespoons minced fresh Italian parsley
2 tablespoons lemon juice
4 tablespoons extra virgin olive oil
1 teaspoon pink Himalayan salt
2 tablespoons minced fresh basil
2 tomatoes, chopped
6 cups arugula

1. Place the chicken breasts between two pieces of parchment paper. Using a meat tenderizer, pound the breasts until they are about ¼ inch thick.
2. In a large bowl, combine the garlic, oregano, thyme, parsley, 1 tablespoon of the lemon juice, 1 tablespoon of the olive oil, and the salt. Using tongs, add the chicken

breasts to the bowl and mix to coat. (Optional: let the coated chicken breasts marinate in the refrigerator for 20 minutes.)

3. In a large skillet, heat 1 tablespoon of the remaining olive oil over medium-high heat. Pan-fry the chicken breasts until cooked through, 3 to 4 minutes per side.

4. In a large salad bowl, add the remaining 2 tablespoons olive oil, 1 tablespoon lemon juice, and the basil. Add the tomatoes and arugula and toss to coat.

5. Plate each chicken breast with half of the salad mixture.

# Coconut Cauliflower Rice with Sweet Coconut Chicken and Broccoli

**MAKES 2 SERVINGS**

You can elevate any family favorite by lowering the sugar content, adding vegetables, and swapping in healthier condiments. This recipe is my favorite childhood teriyaki chicken bowl, elevated.

2 cups broccoli florets

2 tablespoons coconut oil

2 tablespoons coconut milk (or coconut cream)

4 cups frozen or uncooked cauliflower rice

Meat from 1 rotisserie chicken (or 2 baked
    chicken breasts), shredded

2 tablespoons melted ghee

¼ cup coconut aminos

2 tablespoons sesame seeds

2 tablespoons chopped fresh chives

1. Bring 2 inches of water in a large saucepan to a simmer and quick-blanch the broccoli for 4 to 6 minutes, until fork tender. Drain the broccoli and set it aside.

2. In the same pan, combine the coconut oil, coconut milk, and cauliflower rice. Stir-fry over medium heat until the cauliflower rice is done to your liking, 5 to 7 minutes. Add the broccoli and chicken to the pan and cook until warmed through, stirring as needed.

3. In a small bowl, mix the melted ghee, coconut aminos, and sesame seeds. Serve the cauliflower rice in bowls and dress it with the sauce. Garnish with the chives.

# Cowboy Skillet

If you loved Hamburger Helper, this one-pot dinner is for you. It provides an explosion of umami flavor your family will crave, and it's ready in under fifteen minutes.

1 pound ground beef
1 tablespoon smoked paprika
1 tablespoon chili powder
1 tablespoon unsweetened organic ketchup (I like Primal
    Kitchen)
½ tablespoon garlic salt
1 (12-ounce) bag frozen cauliflower rice
1 to 2 cups shredded or finely diced vegetables (optional)
8 cups fresh spinach
2 tablespoons nutritional yeast (optional)

1.  Place the beef in a large skillet and cook over medium-high heat, breaking it into pieces with a wooden spoon, until browned and cooked through, 7 to 10 minutes. Add the paprika, chili powder, ketchup, garlic salt, cauliflower rice, and vegetables (if using) to the meat in the skillet. Stir to combine and cook until heated through, 3 to 4 minutes. Add the spinach and cook until lightly wilted, 1 to 2 minutes.

2.  If you want a cheesy flavor, sprinkle the nutritional yeast on top, then serve.

BODY LOVE A JOURNAL

# Chicken Kale Cobb Snob Salad

**MAKES 2 SERVINGS**

A LeVeque family favorite, this Cobb salad is filling enough to serve for dinner and perfect for leftovers.

## Dressing

½ cup extra virgin olive oil
¼ cup red wine vinegar
Juice of ½ lemon
1 tablespoon gluten-free Worcestershire sauce
1 teaspoon Dijon mustard
Pink Himalayan salt and freshly ground black pepper

## Salad

4 cups chopped kale
1 cooked organic chicken breast, chopped
2 hard-boiled eggs, sliced
2 organic nitrate-free bacon slices, cooked and crumbled
¼ cup chopped cashews
¼ cup shredded carrot (optional)
¼ cup shredded red cabbage (optional)
¼ cup halved cherry tomatoes

1. In a salad bowl, whisk together the dressing ingredients.
2. Add the salad ingredients and toss to coat with the dressing.
3. Divide the salad between two plates and serve.

# Butter-Lettuce-Wrapped Shrimp Tacos

**MAKES 2 TO 4 SERVINGS**

Bring the beach home with these spicy shrimp tacos! They are juicy, crisp, and full of fiber!

1 pound raw wild shrimp, shelled and deveined

1 to 2 tablespoons taco seasoning (for my homemade version, see *Body Love*, page 183)

¼ cup Primal Kitchen mayonnaise (I prefer Primal's mayo because its eggs are pasture-raised, the oil used is avocado, and it contains very little sugar)

Juice of 1 lime

4 cups shredded cabbage (from about ½ cabbage)

2 tablespoons avocado oil or other high-smoke-point oil (see page 30)

1 butter lettuce head, leaves separated

1 avocado, cut into small cubes

¼ cup chopped fresh cilantro

Lime wedges, for serving

1. In a medium bowl, coat the shrimp with the taco seasoning.

2. In a large bowl, mix the mayonnaise with the lime juice and whisk until thinned. Add the cabbage and mix to coat.

3. In a large skillet, heat the oil over medium heat. Add the shrimp and pan-fry until pink and cooked through, 4 to 5 minutes.

4. Place the lettuce leaves on a plate and use them as taco shells, layering in the shrimp, slaw, avocado, and cilantro. Serve with the lime wedges alongside.

# Roasted Black Bean Vegan Burgers

Free of processed protein and loaded with vegetables, this vegan burger will satisfy any carnivore. Make a double batch and freeze the rest for a quick weeknight meal.

1 tablespoon avocado oil

1 tablespoon chili powder

1 tablespoon ground cumin

1½ teaspoons smoked paprika

3 garlic cloves, minced

8 ounces shiitake mushrooms

1 carrot, roughly chopped

1 green bell pepper, roughly chopped

½ yellow onion, finely diced

2 cups canned black beans, drained and rinsed

2 tablespoons unsweetened organic ketchup (I like Primal Kitchen)

½ cup walnuts

¼ cup flax meal

2 cups packed fresh spinach

¼ cup aquafaba, or 2 flax eggs (see *Body Love Every Day* or look online for directions)

8 romaine, butter, or red-leaf lettuce cups

**Toppings of choice:** avocado, tomato, grilled onion, thinly sliced red onion, sautéed sliced mushrooms, fried egg (if you don't need to keep it vegan)

**Condiments of choice**: sugar-free alternatives like Primal Kitchen ketchup, mustard, barbecue sauce, or Thousand Island dressing

1. Preheat the oven to 400°F.
2. In a large bowl, whisk the avocado oil, chili powder, cumin, smoked paprika, and garlic. Add the mushrooms, carrot, green pepper, and onion and toss to coat. Spread the seasoned vegetables on a baking sheet and roast for 20 minutes (flipping them at 10 minutes) to caramelize them and remove most of the water (see Note).
3. Meanwhile, spread the beans on a separate baking sheet and roast them along with the vegetables for 10 minutes, or until they're dried out a bit (some will split open).
4. In a food processor, pulse the roasted vegetables with the ketchup, walnuts, flax meal, and spinach. Take care not to overprocess; you want the veggies in tiny chunks about the size of bread crumbs.
5. In a large bowl, combine the roasted beans, aquafaba, and vegetable-nut mix gently but thoroughly, using your hands. Form the mixture into 4 patties.
6. Pan-fry the patties in a large skillet over medium heat for 4 minutes per side, until warm and set.
7. Wrap each burger in 2 lettuce leaf cups and add your choice of toppings and condiments.

**NOTE:** Removing the water is key! If you don't cook the veggies enough now, the patty mixture will be too wet, disrupting the burger consistency. When in doubt, roughly chop the veggies into 1-inch pieces, or roast longer if needed.

# FAB FOUR SMOOTHIE FORMULA

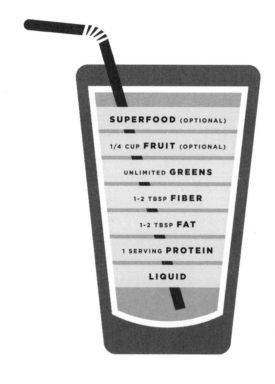

SUPERFOOD (OPTIONAL)

1/4 CUP FRUIT (OPTIONAL)

UNLIMITED GREENS

1-2 TBSP FIBER

1-2 TBSP FAT

1 SERVING PROTEIN

LIQUID

# QUICK REFERENCE CHARTS AND LISTS

Here are a few convenient charts and lists to help you nail your #fab4lifestyle and be well every day!

## HAND SERVING SIZE REFERENCES

You can use the references below to tell easily how much protein, liquid fat, whole food fat, and fiber and greens you should typically include in a meal. Your hand is always handy!

**PROTEIN:** size and thickness of 1 to 2 palms
**LIQUID FAT:** 1 to 2 thumbs (top)
**WHOLE-FOOD FAT:** 1 to 2 thumbs (whole thumb)
**FIBER AND GREENS:** 2 to 4 fists

## HEALTHY OILS LIST/SMOKE POINTS

**High Heat**
Refined Avocado Oil: 520°F
Ghee: 450°F
Pastured Animal Fat (Duck, Tallow, and Lard): 375 to 400°F
Extra Virgin Coconut Oil: 350 to 365°F
Refined Coconut Oil: 450°F

**Light Cooking and Cold Use**
Extra Virgin Avocado Oil: 400°F
Macadamia Oil: 390°F
Extra Virgin Olive Oil: 325 to 375°F
Grass-fed Butter: 300°F

**Cold Use**
Nut and Seed Oils (Almond, Sesame, Hemp, Walnut, Pumpkin, and Flaxseed)

# VEGETABLES AND FRUITS
## THE FIBER RUNDOWN

Wondering what vegetables and fruits to choose every day? Start here for more informed choices!

## Vegetable Nutrition
### Nonstarchy Vegetables
Load your plate with nonstarchy vegetables! These cellular carbohydrates are whole plant foods that are made up of a

combination of starch and/or sugar wrapped in a fiber cell and packed with vitamins, minerals, water, and fiber. Fiber doesn't break down into blood sugar, and needing to be digested slowly to access that sugar and starch helps to support blood sugar balance. Only the starch and sugar components raise blood sugar, and these nonstarchy, low-carb vegetables provide a balanced average of only 5 net grams of carbohydrate per ½ cup cooked or 1 cup raw serving size.

- amaranth or Chinese spinach
- artichokes/artichoke hearts
- asparagus
- bamboo shoots
- beans (green, filet, wax, Italian, yard-long)
- bean sprouts
- broccoli
- Brussels sprouts
- cabbage (green, bok choy, Chinese, Napa, red, savoy)
- carrots
- cauliflower
- celery
- cucumber
- daikon radish
- eggplant
- greens, bitter (collard, kale, mustard, Swiss chard, turnip)

- greens, salad (arugula, chicory, endive, escarole, lettuce, mâche, romaine, radicchio, spinach, watercress)
- hearts of palm
- jicama
- kohlrabi
- leeks
- mushrooms (all types)
- okra
- onions (white, yellow, green, red)
- pea pods/sugar snap peas
- peppers (all types)
- radishes
- squash (yellow summer, zucchini)
- tomato
- turnips
- water chestnuts

**Lightly Starchy Vegetables**

These vegetables are great to incorporate if you are looking to increase your carbohydrate intake gradually without surging blood sugar.

- beets
- squash (butternut, kabocha, spaghetti)
- yams/sweet potatoes

**Starchy/High-Carb Vegetables and Grains**

These foods should be used to support glycogen stores and refuel your muscles post-workout when your muscles are insulin sensitive and ready to store a larger amount of glucose (blood sugar).

- potatoes
- grains (rice, quinoa, amaranth, oats, buckwheat, millet)

## Fruit Nutrition

**Nutrient-Dense Fruit**

When available, opt for nutrient-dense fruits with the highest phytochemical, antioxidant, and fiber levels, like berries.

- blackberries
- blueberries
- raspberries
- strawberries

**Fiber-Rich Fruit**

Enjoy a single serving of fiber-rich fruit.

- apple
- kiwi
- orange
- pear
- stone fruit (peach, plum, apricot, nectarine)

**High-Sugar Fruit**

Keep high-sugar fruits to an appropriate serving size—a small slice or handful.

- banana (opt for a small organic banana)
- cherries
- grapes
- mango
- papaya
- pineapple

# PART II

# CHANGING YOUR MIND-SET

# TIPS AND TRICKS

These are the daily tools I recommend for making sustainable change in your life. Each activity takes work, but it's work that enriches your life and solidifies change. Each tool achieves a different objective: positivity tracking infuses your life with gratitude; anchor appointments ensure you're building and sustaining your healthy lifestyle; and SMART goals help you develop specific and actionable ways to accomplish your goals, grow as an individual, and live your dreams.

# DAILY POSITIVITY TRACKING

Positivity tracking is gratitude with specificity. In this journal, every day you will be tasked to find three specific things to be grateful for. They cannot be vague generalizations, and they cannot repeat. As you start to incorporate this practice into your life, you'll see how beautiful your life becomes—not because it has drastically changed, but because you're experiencing it with a grateful, open heart.

Here are three personal examples of positivity tracking:

- Bash's unstoppable bath-time giggles when he was blowing bubbles into his water cup and the cute way he kept checking to see if I was laughing too.
- Reading a real book today during lunch instead of scrolling through Instagram, and feeling rejuvenated as I returned to the workday in a fresh way.
- Chris's involvement in the family text chain. He goes above and beyond to celebrate everyone else! I just love how special he made my sister feel today about her upcoming delivery and my little niece on the way.

# WEEKLY ANCHOR APPOINTMENTS

Anchors are the weekly appointments you set with yourself that ensure you don't go an entire week without doing what brings you joy, keeps you sane, or makes you better. A weekly religious service is a great example; if you go every week, it's a built-in routine for you, without much anxiety, stress, or effort. You probably aren't forcing yourself to go to morning mass every day, but a once-a-week appointment creates a simple balance with expectation. With health and wellness, we tend to overpromise and under-deliver, and we're either in the routine or out of it. Anchor appointments help to make sure you never fully fall out of a routine.

To develop your anchor appointments, start with what healthy activities you'd like to prioritize in your life. A few examples might be eating more fiber and greens, working out, and prioritizing sleep. Then place a specific "anchor" on the calendar to achieve those priorities. Anchor appointments can't be canceled, and there's never more than one of them booked in a day, so the maximum number you'll ever have on the calendar is seven. I suggest starting slow, with just a few anchor appointments at a time. The objective is to build these behaviors into effortless habits that enrich your life without adding anxiety.

Here are three specific anchor appointments that work for me:

- **MONDAY A.M.:** My Monday morning #fab4smoothie is always a super-green, hydrating, and fiber-rich recipe. It sets the tone for my week and helps me get back in the habit if I had a traditional weekend breakfast.
- **SATURDAY A.M.:** I always attend my 9:30 A.M. yoga class. This me time is a negotiated weekend hour to myself in which my husband, Chris, watches our son, Bash. As an entrepreneur, I need help to unwind, and this sets the tone for my weekend, keeping me moving and ensuring that work obligations never get in the way.
- **SUNDAY NIGHT:** I set a 9 P.M. no-screens bedtime for Sunday night. This helps me start the week fresh rather than stay up late streaming the next bingeworthy show. This "in-bed" anchor is paramount for my ability to eat clean, work out with intensity, and efficiently complete work tasks.

Don't be afraid to ask for help! It's better to get started with support than not to start at all, so if your goal is to get active, find an accountability partner, schedule your classes in advance, or hire a trainer for the first few weeks to help ensure your commitment to the weekly anchor appointment.

# MONTHLY SMART GOALS

To keep my clients' goals realistic and attainable, we set one SMART goal at a time. I often rely on the framework that I talked about in *Body Love*.

"**SMART**" stands for

- **S**pecific: be specific in setting the goal you want to achieve. This could be something like "I'll make a Fab Four smoothie every day for the next three weeks before eleven A.M."
- **M**easurable: set a metric to quantify the success of the outcome. That's simple: twenty-one smoothies in twenty-one days.
- **A**chievable: challenge yourself, but make sure you're able to achieve your goal. It might not be realistic to eat Fab Four meals at every meal at first, so start with breakfast.
- **R**elevant: keep smaller goals relevant to higher goals. If your larger goal is to increase energy, it starts with balancing your blood sugar at each meal—so let's start with the most important one, breakfast!
- **T**imebound: set a date for when you want to achieve your goal. Once it's completed, you can recommit (and adjust if necessary). If you start on January 1, your end date is January 21.

Every successfully completed SMART goal is a win! You're showing yourself that you're in control of your life and have follow-through, and that relationship with goals—including nutrition-related goals—can breed confidence. This monthly ritual requires you to be surgical about your approach, but it greatly increases the likelihood of completion.

# SAMPLE TRACKING CHARTS

You'll be filling in daily, weekly, and monthly tracking charts throughout the 90 days that follow. These sample charts offer you some guidance on how to fill them in.

# Sample Daily Expression

**Week 1/Date:** *November 2*

BODY LOVE A JOURNAL

## HIT LIST

Write down three top priorities of the day that will move the ball on your goals:

1. *Pick up groceries*

2. *Confirm January doctor's appointments*

3. *Send Hannah session notes via email*

## HYDRATION

Check off one droplet for each 8 ounces water you consume today.

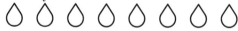

## MOVEMENT

What have I done today to move my body?

*yoga class, 30-minute morning walk*

# MEALS

**BREAKFAST:** Spa Smoothie

- ☐ Protein: BWBK Vanilla Protein
- ☐ Fat: Avocado
- ☐ Fiber: Chia + 1 teaspoon acacia
- ☐ Greens: Spinach, cucumber, and mint

**LUNCH:** Chopped Salad

- ☐ Protein: Chicken
- ☐ Fat: Tahini dressing
- ☐ Fiber: Radish, zucchini, tomato, cucumber
- ☐ Greens: Romaine and microgreens

**DINNER:** Cowboy Skillet

- ☐ Protein: Ground beef
- ☐ Fat: Avocado oil
- ☐ Fiber: Cauliflower rice
- ☐ Greens: Spinach

Write down three new and specific things you are grateful for today:

1. Tonight's sunset was magical. It closed out the workday, and the rest of the evening was spent reading.

2. A little ACV in my water this afternoon, and that refreshing cup of cold water was delightful. I need to create a trigger for that habit—I downed my water today! Whoop!

3. Read your IG comments and feel the love. This is your why! Juli lost 50 pounds with the #fab4smoothie and kept it off, then three other ladies commented on her post saying they all lost significant amounts too.

Write your thoughts and emotions out of your head and body and onto the page. Let go.

Feeling super distracted and anxious for tomorrow's presentation and am wanting all the treats. Oy vey. These are just emotional cravings. All this overthinking is making me crazy. Time to breathe or flow. You are just nervous because you care, not because you are underprepared. You've got this!

# Sample Weekly Planning

## SMOOTHIE INSPO

Write down three fun smoothie ideas for the next week:

1. *Icy FAB-uccino*

2. *Spa Smoothie*

3. _____

## #FAB4SMOOTHIE GROCERY LIST

- ☐ Liquid
    - ☐ Almond milk
    - ☑ *Macadamia nut milk*
- ☐ Protein
    - ☑ Vanilla
    - ☐ Chocolate
    - ☐ _____
- ☐ Fat
    - ☑ Avocado

47

- ☐ Nut Butter _____
- ☐ _____

☐ Fiber _____
- ☑ Chia _____
- ☐ Flax _____
- ☐ Fiber Powders (acacia, psyllium, husk) _____
- ☐ _____

☐ Greens _____
- ☑ Fresh _____
- ☐ Frozen _____

☐ Fruit _____
- ☐ Fresh _____
    - ☐ Berries _____
    - ☐ Citrus _____
- ☑ Tropical _____
- ☐ Frozen _____
    - ☐ Berries _____
    - ☐ _____

## WEEKLY MEAL PREP

Write down three great meal ideas for the next week:

1. *Shrimp tacos*

2. *Italian chicken*

3. *Cobb salad*

Which bulk protein do you want to use for your lunches?

*Salmon salad and hard-boiled eggs*

## FAB FOUR GROCERY LIST

☐ Protein

    ☐ *1 pound wild shrimp*

    ☐ *4 chicken breasts*

    ☐ *Dozen eggs*

    ☐ *Wild salmon*

☐ Fat

    ☐ Cooking Oils *Avocado and olive*

    ☐ Dressing *Cobb*

    ☐ Dip *Pesto (nuts, garlic, basil)*

- ☐ Nonstarchy Fiber-Rich Vegetables

  - ☐ _Cabbage and radicchio (or slaw mix)_
  - ☐ _Tomatoes_
  - ☐ _Cucumber_
  - ☐ _Broccoli_
  - ☐ _Radish_
  - ☐ _Brussels sprouts_

- ☐ Greens

  - ☐ Salad Greens _Butter lettuce, romaine, arugula_
  - ☐ Herbs _Basil_

- ☐ Starch (one per week of savory and sweet)

  - ☐ Savory _Sweet potato cubes as croutons for the Cobb!_
  - ☐ Sweet _Freezer fudge_
  - ☐

## ANCHOR APPOINTMENTS

**MONDAY**  *Fab Four Smoothie every Monday before 11 a.m.*

**TUESDAY**

**WEDNESDAY**  *HIIT with Lisa at 5 p.m.*

**THURSDAY**

**FRIDAY**

**SATURDAY**  *No work. Read for an hour with coffee before starting the day.*

**SUNDAY**

# Sample Monthly Manifestation

**Month:** _November_

## GO IN

Identify self-limiting beliefs and emotional patterns holding you back.

_It's too late for me!_

_I'll always emotionally eat._

## LET GO

Take a moment to forgive yourself, release resentment, and erase regrets. It's time to let go of these beliefs and move forward.

_I am sad, and sorry for being so hard on myself and my body. I restrict to be perfect, and when things go wrong, I binge and feel like a failure all over again. I am doing this to myself, I am creating this pressure. With more flexibility, I know I can change and give my body a break._

With nothing holding you back, visualize what your life would look like in a month, a year, five years, and ten years from now and write it down, being as specific as possible.

*In one month, I will have enrolled in school. In five years, I'll be a working graphic designer with a thriving brand consulting business, a beautiful website, and happy customers.*

*In ten years, I will have bought my first house and hired at least one employee and my work will have been featured or published in press.*

*In one month, I will have loved on my body by eating consistently and enjoyed a few desserts without regret. In five years, I will feel at peace with my body, will focus on fueling it with good food, and will have quieted my inner perfectionist. In ten years, I will have a garden, make my favorite meals from scratch, and share them with friends. I will taste, enjoy, and celebrate food.*

Using the SMART goals framework on page 41, be specific about the repeatable and actionable steps you plan to take this month.

1.  My goal is to _eat healthier,_ so I'll _meal prep light every Sunday_ for _2_ (days/weeks/(months)) by _2 p.m._ (time) to _support my goal and have healthy options to reach for._

2.  My goal is to _____ so I'll _____ for _____ (days/weeks/months) by _____ (time) to _____.

BODY LOVE A JOURNAL

54

# DAILY EXPRESSION, WEEKLY PREPARATION, AND MONTHLY MANIFESTATION TRACKING CHARTS

# Monthly Manifestation

**Month:** _____

Identify self-limiting beliefs and emotional patterns
holding you back.

Take a moment to forgive yourself, release resentment,
and erase regrets. It's time to let go of these beliefs and
move forward.

TRACKING CHARTS

57

## MANIFEST MAGIC

With nothing holding you back, visualize what your life would look like in a month, a year, five years, and ten years from now and write it down, being as specific as possible.

## MONTHLY SMART GOALS

Using the SMART goals framework on page 41, be specific about the repeatable and actionable steps you plan to take this month.

1. _____

2. _____

3. _____

# Weekly Planning

**Week 1:** _____

## SMOOTHIE INSPO

Write down three fun smoothie ideas for the next week:

1. _____

2. _____

3. _____

## #FAB4SMOOTHIE GROCERY LIST

☐ Liquid _____

    ☐ Nut Milk _____

    ☐ _____

☐ Protein _____

    ☐ Vanilla _____

    ☐ Chocolate _____

    ☐ _____

☐ Fat _____

    ☐ Avocado _____

    ☐ Nut Butter _____

    ☐ Coconut _____

    ☐ Healthy Oils _____

    ☐ _____

☐ Fiber _____

    ☐ Chia _____

    ☐ Flax _____

    ☐ Fiber Powders (acacia, psyllium husk) _____

☐ Greens _____

    ☐ Fresh _____

    ☐ Frozen _____

☐ Fruit _____

    ☐ Fresh _____

        ☐ Berries _____

        ☐ Citrus _____

        ☐ Tropical _____

    ☐ Frozen _____

        ☐ Berries _____

## WEEKLY MEAL PREP

Write down three great meal ideas for the next week:

1. _____

2. _____

3. _____

Which bulk protein do you want to use for your lunches?

_____

## FAB FOUR GROCERY LIST

☐ Protein

  ☐ _____

  ☐ _____

  ☐ _____

☐ Fat

  ☐ Cooking Oils _____

  ☐ Dressing _____

  ☐ Dip _____

☐ Nonstarchy Fiber-Rich Vegetables

   ☐ _____

   ☐ _____

   ☐ _____

   ☐ _____

☐ Greens

   ☐ Salad Greens _____

   ☐ Herbs _____

☐ Starch (one per week of savory and sweet)

   ☐ Savory _____

   ☐ Sweet _____

## ANCHOR APPOINTMENTS

**MONDAY**

**TUESDAY**

**WEDNESDAY**

**THURSDAY**

**FRIDAY**

**SATURDAY**

**SUNDAY**

# Daily Expression

## Week 1/Date: _____

### HIT LIST

Write down three top priorities of the day that will move the ball on your goals:

1. _____

2. _____

3. _____

### HYDRATION

Check off one droplet for each 8 ounces water you consume today.

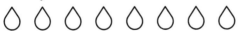

### MOVEMENT

What have I done today to move my body?

## MEALS

**BREAKFAST:** _____

☐ Protein: _____

☐ Fat: _____

☐ Fiber: _____

☐ Greens: _____


**LUNCH:** _____

☐ Protein: _____

☐ Fat: _____

☐ Fiber: _____

☐ Greens: _____


**DINNER:** _____

☐ Protein: _____

☐ Fat: _____

☐ Fiber: _____

☐ Greens: _____

## POSITIVITY TRACKING

Write down three new and specific things you are grateful for today:

*1.*

*2.*

*3.*

## PARKING LOT

Write your thoughts and emotions out of your head and body and onto the page. Let go.

# Daily Expression

## Week 1/Date: _____

### HIT LIST

Write down three top priorities of the day that will move the ball on your goals:

1. _____

2. _____

3. _____

### HYDRATION

Check off one droplet for each 8 ounces water you consume today.

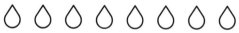

### MOVEMENT

What have I done today to move my body?

# MEALS

**BREAKFAST:** _____

☐ Protein: _____

☐ Fat: _____

☐ Fiber: _____

☐ Greens: _____


**LUNCH:** _____

☐ Protein: _____

☐ Fat: _____

☐ Fiber: _____

☐ Greens: _____


**DINNER:** _____

☐ Protein: _____

☐ Fat: _____

☐ Fiber: _____

☐ Greens: _____

TRACKING CHARTS

67

Write down three new and specific things you are grateful for today:

1.

2.

3.

Write your thoughts and emotions out of your head and body and onto the page. Let go.

BODY LOVE A JOURNAL

# Daily Expression

**Week 1/Date:** _____

## HIT LIST

Write down three top priorities of the day that will move the ball on your goals:

*1.* _____

*2.* _____

*3.* _____

## HYDRATION

Check off one droplet for each 8 ounces water you consume today.

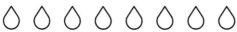

## MOVEMENT

What have I done today to move my body?

## MEALS

**BREAKFAST:** _____

☐ Protein: _____

☐ Fat: _____

☐ Fiber: _____

☐ Greens: _____

**LUNCH:** _____

☐ Protein: _____

☐ Fat: _____

☐ Fiber: _____

☐ Greens: _____

**DINNER:** _____

☐ Protein: _____

☐ Fat: _____

☐ Fiber: _____

☐ Greens: _____

## POSITIVITY TRACKING

Write down three new and specific things you are grateful for today:

*1.*

*2.*

*3.*

## PARKING LOT

Write your thoughts and emotions out of your head and body and onto the page. Let go.

# Daily Expression

## Week 1/Date: _____

**HIT LIST**

Write down three top priorities of the day that will move the ball on your goals:

*1.* _____

*2.* _____

*3.* _____

**HYDRATION**

Check off one droplet for each 8 ounces water you consume today.

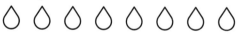

**MOVEMENT**

What have I done today to move my body?

BODY LOVE A JOURNAL

## MEALS

**BREAKFAST:** _____

☐ Protein: _____

☐ Fat: _____

☐ Fiber: _____

☐ Greens: _____


**LUNCH:** _____

☐ Protein: _____

☐ Fat: _____

☐ Fiber: _____

☐ Greens: _____


**DINNER:** _____

☐ Protein: _____

☐ Fat: _____

☐ Fiber: _____

☐ Greens: _____

TRACKING CHARTS

73

Write down three new and specific things you are grateful for today:

1.

2.

3.

Write your thoughts and emotions out of your head and body and onto the page. Let go.

BODY LOVE A JOURNAL

# Daily Expression

## Week 1/Date: _____

### HIT LIST

Write down three top priorities of the day that will move the ball on your goals:

1. _____

2. _____

3. _____

### HYDRATION

Check off one droplet for each 8 ounces water you consume today.

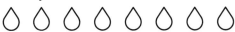

### MOVEMENT

What have I done today to move my body?

## MEALS

**BREAKFAST:** _____

- ☐ Protein: _____
- ☐ Fat: _____
- ☐ Fiber: _____
- ☐ Greens: _____

**LUNCH:** _____

- ☐ Protein: _____
- ☐ Fat: _____
- ☐ Fiber: _____
- ☐ Greens: _____

**DINNER:** _____

- ☐ Protein: _____
- ☐ Fat: _____
- ☐ Fiber: _____
- ☐ Greens: _____

## POSITIVITY TRACKING

Write down three new and specific things you are grateful for today:

1.

2.

3.

## PARKING LOT

Write your thoughts and emotions out of your head and body and onto the page. Let go.

# Daily Expression

## Week 1/Date: _____

**HIT LIST**

Write down three top priorities of the day that will move the ball on your goals:

1. _____

2. _____

3. _____

**HYDRATION**

Check off one droplet for each 8 ounces water you consume today.

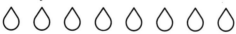

**MOVEMENT**

What have I done today to move my body?

## MEALS

**BREAKFAST:** _____

☐ Protein: _____

☐ Fat: _____

☐ Fiber: _____

☐ Greens: _____


**LUNCH:** _____

☐ Protein: _____

☐ Fat: _____

☐ Fiber: _____

☐ Greens: _____


**DINNER:** _____

☐ Protein: _____

☐ Fat: _____

☐ Fiber: _____

☐ Greens: _____

TRACKING CHARTS

Write down three new and specific things you are grateful for today:

1.

2.

3.

## PARKING LOT

Write your thoughts and emotions out of your head and body and onto the page. Let go.

# Daily Expression

## Week 1/Date: _____

### HIT LIST

Write down three top priorities of the day that will move the ball on your goals:

1. _____

2. _____

3. _____

### HYDRATION

Check off one droplet for each 8 ounces water you consume today.

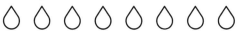

### MOVEMENT

What have I done today to move my body?

## MEALS

**BREAKFAST:** _____

☐  Protein: _____

☐  Fat: _____

☐  Fiber: _____

☐  Greens: _____


**LUNCH:** _____

☐  Protein: _____

☐  Fat: _____

☐  Fiber: _____

☐  Greens: _____


**DINNER:** _____

☐  Protein: _____

☐  Fat: _____

☐  Fiber: _____

☐  Greens: _____

## POSITIVITY TRACKING

Write down three new and specific things you are grateful for today:

*1.*

*2.*

*3.*

## PARKING LOT

Write your thoughts and emotions out of your head and body and onto the page. Let go.

# Weekly Planning

**Week 2:** _____

## SMOOTHIE INSPO

Write down three fun smoothie ideas for the next week:

*1.* _____

*2.* _____

*3.* _____

## #FAB4SMOOTHIE GROCERY LIST

☐ Liquid _____

    ☐ Nut Milk _____

    ☐ _____

☐ Protein _____

    ☐ Vanilla _____

    ☐ Chocolate _____

    ☐ _____

☐ Fat _____

   ☐   Avocado _____

   ☐   Nut Butter _____

   ☐   Coconut _____

   ☐   Healthy Oils _____

   ☐   _____

☐ Fiber _____

   ☐   Chia _____

   ☐   Flax _____

   ☐   Fiber Powders (acacia, psyllium husk) _____

☐ Greens _____

   ☐   Fresh _____

   ☐   Frozen _____

☐ Fruit _____

   ☐   Fresh _____

      ☐   Berries _____

      ☐   Citrus _____

      ☐   Tropical _____

   ☐   Frozen _____

      ☐   Berries _____

## WEEKLY MEAL PREP

Write down three great meal ideas for the next week:

1. _____

2. _____

3. _____

Which bulk protein do you want to use for your lunches?

_____

## FAB FOUR GROCERY LIST

☐ Protein

   ☐ _____

   ☐ _____

   ☐ _____

☐ Fat

   ☐ Cooking Oils _____

   ☐ Dressing _____

   ☐ Dip _____

☐ Nonstarchy Fiber-Rich Vegetables

    ☐ _____

    ☐ _____

    ☐ _____

    ☐ _____

☐ Greens

    ☐ Salad Greens _____

    ☐ Herbs _____

☐ Starch (one per week of savory and sweet)

    ☐ Savory _____

    ☐ Sweet _____

## ANCHOR APPOINTMENTS

**MONDAY**

**TUESDAY**

**WEDNESDAY**

**THURSDAY**

**FRIDAY**

**SATURDAY**

**SUNDAY**

# Daily Expression

## Week 2/Date: _____

### HIT LIST

Write down three top priorities of the day that will move the ball on your goals:

1. _____

2. _____

3. _____

### HYDRATION

Check off one droplet for each 8 ounces water you consume today.

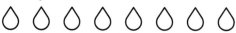

### MOVEMENT

What have I done today to move my body?

## MEALS

**BREAKFAST:** _____

☐ Protein: _____

☐ Fat: _____

☐ Fiber: _____

☐ Greens: _____


**LUNCH:** _____

☐ Protein: _____

☐ Fat: _____

☐ Fiber: _____

☐ Greens: _____


**DINNER:** _____

☐ Protein: _____

☐ Fat: _____

☐ Fiber: _____

☐ Greens: _____

TRACKING CHARTS

## POSITIVITY TRACKING

Write down three new and specific things you are grateful for today:

1.

2.

3.

## PARKING LOT

Write your thoughts and emotions out of your head and body and onto the page. Let go.

# Daily Expression

## Week 2/Date: _____

### HIT LIST

Write down three top priorities of the day that will move the ball on your goals:

1. _____

2. _____

3. _____

### HYDRATION

Check off one droplet for each 8 ounces water you consume today.

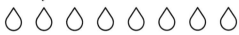

### MOVEMENT

What have I done today to move my body?

## MEALS

**BREAKFAST:** _____

☐ Protein: _____

☐ Fat: _____

☐ Fiber: _____

☐ Greens: _____

**LUNCH:** _____

☐ Protein: _____

☐ Fat: _____

☐ Fiber: _____

☐ Greens: _____

**DINNER:** _____

☐ Protein: _____

☐ Fat: _____

☐ Fiber: _____

☐ Greens: _____

## POSITIVITY TRACKING

Write down three new and specific things you are grateful for today:

1.

2.

3.

## PARKING LOT

Write your thoughts and emotions out of your head and body and onto the page. Let go.

# Daily Expression

## Week 2/Date: _____

### HIT LIST

Write down three top priorities of the day that will move the ball on your goals:

*1.* _____

*2.* _____

*3.* _____

### HYDRATION

Check off one droplet for each 8 ounces water you consume today.

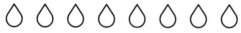

### MOVEMENT

What have I done today to move my body?

## MEALS

**BREAKFAST:** _____

☐ Protein: _____

☐ Fat: _____

☐ Fiber: _____

☐ Greens: _____


**LUNCH:** _____

☐ Protein: _____

☐ Fat: _____

☐ Fiber: _____

☐ Greens: _____


**DINNER:** _____

☐ Protein: _____

☐ Fat: _____

☐ Fiber: _____

☐ Greens: _____

TRACKING CHARTS

## POSITIVITY TRACKING

Write down three new and specific things you are grateful for today:

1.



2.



3.



## PARKING LOT

Write your thoughts and emotions out of your head and body and onto the page. Let go.

# Daily Expression

**Week 2/Date:** _____

## HIT LIST

Write down three top priorities of the day that will move
the ball on your goals:

*1.* _____

*2.* _____

*3.* _____

## HYDRATION

Check off one droplet for each 8 ounces water you
consume today.

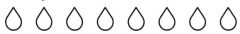

## MOVEMENT

What have I done today to move my body?

97

## MEALS

**BREAKFAST:** _____

☐ Protein: _____

☐ Fat: _____

☐ Fiber: _____

☐ Greens: _____


**LUNCH:** _____

☐ Protein: _____

☐ Fat: _____

☐ Fiber: _____

☐ Greens: _____


**DINNER:** _____

☐ Protein: _____

☐ Fat: _____

☐ Fiber: _____

☐ Greens: _____

## POSITIVITY TRACKING

Write down three new and specific things you are grateful for today:

1.

2.

3.

## PARKING LOT

Write your thoughts and emotions out of your head and body and onto the page. Let go.

# Daily Expression

## Week 2/Date: _____

### HIT LIST

Write down three top priorities of the day that will move
the ball on your goals:

1. _____

2. _____

3. _____

### HYDRATION

Check off one droplet for each 8 ounces water you
consume today.

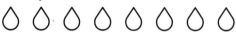

### MOVEMENT

What have I done today to move my body?

## MEALS

**BREAKFAST:** _____

☐ Protein: _____

☐ Fat: _____

☐ Fiber: _____

☐ Greens: _____


**LUNCH:** _____

☐ Protein: _____

☐ Fat: _____

☐ Fiber: _____

☐ Greens: _____


**DINNER:** _____

☐ Protein: _____

☐ Fat: _____

☐ Fiber: _____

☐ Greens: _____

TRACKING CHARTS

Write down three new and specific things you are grateful for today:

1.

2.

3.

**PARKING LOT**

Write your thoughts and emotions out of your head and body and onto the page. Let go.

# Daily Expression

## Week 2/Date: _____

### HIT LIST

Write down three top priorities of the day that will move the ball on your goals:

1. _____

2. _____

3. _____

### HYDRATION

Check off one droplet for each 8 ounces water you consume today.

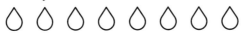

### MOVEMENT

What have I done today to move my body?

## MEALS

**BREAKFAST:** _____

☐  Protein: _____

☐  Fat: _____

☐  Fiber: _____

☐  Greens: _____


**LUNCH:** _____

☐  Protein: _____

☐  Fat: _____

☐  Fiber: _____

☐  Greens: _____


**DINNER:** _____

☐  Protein: _____

☐  Fat: _____

☐  Fiber: _____

☐  Greens: _____

## POSITIVITY TRACKING

Write down three new and specific things you are grateful for today:

1.

2.

3.

## PARKING LOT

Write your thoughts and emotions out of your head and body and onto the page. Let go.

# Daily Expression

### Week 2/Date: _____

## HIT LIST

Write down three top priorities of the day that will move the ball on your goals:

1. _____

2. _____

3. _____

## HYDRATION

Check off one droplet for each 8 ounces water you consume today.

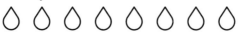

## MOVEMENT

What have I done today to move my body?

## MEALS

**BREAKFAST:** _____

☐ Protein: _____

☐ Fat: _____

☐ Fiber: _____

☐ Greens: _____


**LUNCH:** _____

☐ Protein: _____

☐ Fat: _____

☐ Fiber: _____

☐ Greens: _____


**DINNER:** _____

☐ Protein: _____

☐ Fat: _____

☐ Fiber: _____

☐ Greens: _____

TRACKING CHARTS

## POSITIVITY TRACKING

Write down three new and specific things you are grateful for today:

1.

2.

3.

## PARKING LOT

Write your thoughts and emotions out of your head and body and onto the page. Let go.

# Weekly Planning

**Week 3:** _____

## SMOOTHIE INSPO

Write down three fun smoothie ideas for the next week:

*1.* _____

*2.* _____

*3.* _____

## #FAB4SMOOTHIE GROCERY LIST

☐ Liquid _____

    ☐   Nut Milk _____

    ☐   _____

☐ Protein _____

    ☐   Vanilla _____

    ☐   Chocolate _____

    ☐   _____

- ☐ Fat _____
  - ☐ Avocado _____
  - ☐ Nut Butter _____
  - ☐ Coconut _____
  - ☐ Healthy Oils _____
  - ☐ _____
- ☐ Fiber _____
  - ☐ Chia _____
  - ☐ Flax _____
  - ☐ Fiber Powders (acacia, psyllium husk) _____
- ☐ Greens _____
  - ☐ Fresh _____
  - ☐ Frozen _____
- ☐ Fruit _____
  - ☐ Fresh _____
    - ☐ Berries _____
    - ☐ Citrus _____
    - ☐ Tropical _____
  - ☐ Frozen _____
    - ☐ Berries _____

Write down three great meal ideas for the next week:

1. _____

2. _____

3. _____

Which bulk protein do you want to use for your lunches?

_____

**FAB FOUR GROCERY LIST**

☐ Protein

    ☐ _____

    ☐ _____

    ☐ _____

☐ Fat

    ☐ Cooking Oils _____

    ☐ Dressing _____

    ☐ Dip _____

☐ Nonstarchy Fiber-Rich Vegetables

    ☐ _____

    ☐ _____

    ☐ _____

    ☐ _____

☐ Greens

    ☐ Salad Greens _____

    ☐ Herbs _____

☐ Starch (one per week of savory and sweet)

    ☐ Savory _____

    ☐ Sweet _____

## ANCHOR APPOINTMENTS

**MONDAY**

**TUESDAY**

**WEDNESDAY**

**THURSDAY**

**FRIDAY**

**SATURDAY**

**SUNDAY**

# Daily Expression

**Week 3/Date:** _____

## HIT LIST

Write down three top priorities of the day that will move the ball on your goals:

*1.* _____

*2.* _____

*3.* _____

## HYDRATION

Check off one droplet for each 8 ounces water you consume today.

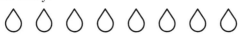

## MOVEMENT

What have I done today to move my body?

## MEALS

**BREAKFAST:** _____

☐ Protein: _____

☐ Fat: _____

☐ Fiber: _____

☐ Greens: _____

**LUNCH:** _____

☐ Protein: _____

☐ Fat: _____

☐ Fiber: _____

☐ Greens: _____

**DINNER:** _____

☐ Protein: _____

☐ Fat: _____

☐ Fiber: _____

☐ Greens: _____

## POSITIVITY TRACKING

Write down three new and specific things you are grateful for today:

*1.*

*2.*

*3.*

.

## PARKING LOT

Write your thoughts and emotions out of your head and body and onto the page. Let go.

# Daily Expression

## Week 3/Date: _____

### HIT LIST

Write down three top priorities of the day that will move the ball on your goals:

1. _____

2. _____

3. _____

### HYDRATION

Check off one droplet for each 8 ounces water you consume today.

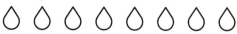

### MOVEMENT

What have I done today to move my body?

## MEALS

**BREAKFAST:** _____

☐ Protein: _____

☐ Fat: _____

☐ Fiber: _____

☐ Greens: _____


**LUNCH:** _____

☐ Protein: _____

☐ Fat: _____

☐ Fiber: _____

☐ Greens: _____


**DINNER:** _____

☐ Protein: _____

☐ Fat: _____

☐ Fiber: _____

☐ Greens: _____

## POSITIVITY TRACKING

Write down three new and specific things you are grateful for today:

1.

2.

3.

## PARKING LOT

Write your thoughts and emotions out of your head and body and onto the page. Let go.

# Daily Expression

**Week 3/Date:** _____

## HIT LIST

Write down three top priorities of the day that will move the ball on your goals:

1. _____

2. _____

3. _____

## HYDRATION

Check off one droplet for each 8 ounces water you consume today.

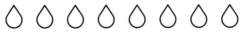

## MOVEMENT

What have I done today to move my body?

## MEALS

**BREAKFAST:** _____

☐ Protein: _____

☐ Fat: _____

☐ Fiber: _____

☐ Greens: _____


**LUNCH:** _____

☐ Protein: _____

☐ Fat: _____

☐ Fiber: _____

☐ Greens: _____


**DINNER:** _____

☐ Protein: _____

☐ Fat: _____

☐ Fiber: _____

☐ Greens: _____

## POSITIVITY TRACKING

Write down three new and specific things you are grateful for today:

1.

2.

3.

## PARKING LOT

Write your thoughts and emotions out of your head and body and onto the page. Let go.

# Daily Expression

## Week 3/Date: _____

### HIT LIST

Write down three top priorities of the day that will move the ball on your goals:

1. _____

2. _____

3. _____

### HYDRATION

Check off one droplet for each 8 ounces water you consume today.

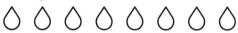

### MOVEMENT

What have I done today to move my body?

## MEALS

**BREAKFAST:** _____

☐ Protein: _____

☐ Fat: _____

☐ Fiber: _____

☐ Greens: _____


**LUNCH:** _____

☐ Protein: _____

☐ Fat: _____

☐ Fiber: _____

☐ Greens: _____


**DINNER:** _____

☐ Protein: _____

☐ Fat: _____

☐ Fiber: _____

☐ Greens: _____

TRACKING CHARTS

## POSITIVITY TRACKING

Write down three new and specific things you are grateful for today:

1.

2.

3.

## PARKING LOT

Write your thoughts and emotions out of your head and body and onto the page. Let go.

# Daily Expression

## Week 3/Date: _____

**HIT LIST**

Write down three top priorities of the day that will move the ball on your goals:

*1.* _____

*2.* _____

*3.* _____

**HYDRATION**

Check off one droplet for each 8 ounces water you consume today.

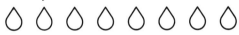

**MOVEMENT**

What have I done today to move my body?

## MEALS

**BREAKFAST:** _____

☐ Protein: _____

☐ Fat: _____

☐ Fiber: _____

☐ Greens: _____


**LUNCH:** _____

☐ Protein: _____

☐ Fat: _____

☐ Fiber: _____

☐ Greens: _____


**DINNER:** _____

☐ Protein: _____

☐ Fat: _____

☐ Fiber: _____

☐ Greens: _____

## POSITIVITY TRACKING

Write down three new and specific things you are grateful for today:

1.

2.

3.

## PARKING LOT

Write your thoughts and emotions out of your head and body and onto the page. Let go.

# Daily Expression

### HIT LIST

Write down three top priorities of the day that will move the ball on your goals:

1. _____

2. _____

3. _____

### HYDRATION

Check off one droplet for each 8 ounces water you consume today.

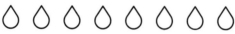

### MOVEMENT

What have I done today to move my body?

## MEALS

**BREAKFAST:** _____

☐ Protein: _____

☐ Fat: _____

☐ Fiber: _____

☐ Greens: _____


**LUNCH:** _____

☐ Protein: _____

☐ Fat: _____

☐ Fiber: _____

☐ Greens: _____


**DINNER:** _____

☐ Protein: _____

☐ Fat: _____

☐ Fiber: _____

☐ Greens: _____

## POSITIVITY TRACKING

Write down three new and specific things you are grateful for today:

1.

2.

3.

## PARKING LOT

Write your thoughts and emotions out of your head and body and onto the page. Let go.

# Daily Expression

**Week 3/Date:** _____

## HIT LIST

Write down three top priorities of the day that will move the ball on your goals:

1. _____

2. _____

3. _____

## HYDRATION

Check off one droplet for each 8 ounces water you consume today.

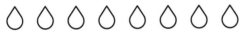

## MOVEMENT

What have I done today to move my body?

## MEALS

**BREAKFAST:** _____

☐ Protein: _____

☐ Fat: _____

☐ Fiber: _____

☐ Greens: _____


**LUNCH:** _____

☐ Protein: _____

☐ Fat: _____

☐ Fiber: _____

☐ Greens: _____


**DINNER:** _____

☐ Protein: _____

☐ Fat: _____

☐ Fiber: _____

☐ Greens: _____

## POSITIVITY TRACKING

Write down three new and specific things you are grateful for today:

1.

2.

3.

## PARKING LOT

Write your thoughts and emotions out of your head and body and onto the page. Let go.

# Weekly Planning

### SMOOTHIE INSPO

Write down three fun smoothie ideas for the next week:

*1.* _____

*2.* _____

*3.* _____

### #FAB4SMOOTHIE GROCERY LIST

☐ Liquid _____

   ☐ Nut Milk _____

   ☐ _____

☐ Protein _____

   ☐ Vanilla _____

   ☐ Chocolate _____

   ☐ _____

☐ Fat _____

    ☐ Avocado _____

    ☐ Nut Butter _____

    ☐ Coconut _____

    ☐ Healthy Oils _____

    ☐ _____

☐ Fiber _____

    ☐ Chia _____

    ☐ Flax _____

    ☐ Fiber Powders (acacia, psyllium husk) _____

☐ Greens _____

    ☐ Fresh _____

    ☐ Frozen _____

☐ Fruit _____

    ☐ Fresh _____

        ☐ Berries _____

        ☐ Citrus _____

        ☐ Tropical _____

    ☐ Frozen _____

        ☐ Berries _____

## WEEKLY MEAL PREP

Write down three great meal ideas for the next week:

1. _____

2. _____

3. _____

Which bulk protein do you want to use for your lunches?

_____

## FAB FOUR GROCERY LIST

☐ Protein

    ☐ _____

    ☐ _____

    ☐ _____

☐ Fat

    ☐ Cooking Oils _____

    ☐ Dressing _____

    ☐ Dip _____

☐ Nonstarchy Fiber-Rich Vegetables

    ☐ _____

    ☐ _____

    ☐ _____

    ☐ _____

☐ Greens

    ☐ Salad Greens _____

    ☐ Herbs _____

☐ Starch (one per week of savory and sweet)

    ☐ Savory _____

    ☐ Sweet _____

## ANCHOR APPOINTMENTS

**MONDAY**

**TUESDAY**

**WEDNESDAY**

**THURSDAY**

**FRIDAY**

**SATURDAY**

**SUNDAY**

# Daily Expression

**HIT LIST**

Write down three top priorities of the day that will move the ball on your goals:

1. _____

2. _____

3. _____

**HYDRATION**

Check off one droplet for each 8 ounces water you consume today.

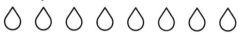

**MOVEMENT**

What have I done today to move my body?

BODY LOVE A JOURNAL

## MEALS

**BREAKFAST:** _____

☐ Protein: _____

☐ Fat: _____

☐ Fiber: _____

☐ Greens: _____


**LUNCH:** _____

☐ Protein: _____

☐ Fat: _____

☐ Fiber: _____

☐ Greens: _____


**DINNER:** _____

☐ Protein: _____

☐ Fat: _____

☐ Fiber: _____

☐ Greens: _____

TRACKING CHARTS

Write down three new and specific things you are grateful for today:

1.

2.

3.

**PARKING LOT**

Write your thoughts and emotions out of your head and body and onto the page. Let go.

# Daily Expression

**Week 4/Date:** _____

### HIT LIST

Write down three top priorities of the day that will move the ball on your goals:

*1.* _____

*2.* _____

*3.* _____

### HYDRATION

Check off one droplet for each 8 ounces water you consume today.

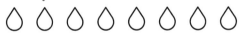

### MOVEMENT

What have I done today to move my body?

141

## MEALS

**BREAKFAST:** _____

- ☐ Protein: _____
- ☐ Fat: _____
- ☐ Fiber: _____
- ☐ Greens: _____

**LUNCH:** _____

- ☐ Protein: _____
- ☐ Fat: _____
- ☐ Fiber: _____
- ☐ Greens: _____

**DINNER:** _____

- ☐ Protein: _____
- ☐ Fat: _____
- ☐ Fiber: _____
- ☐ Greens: _____

## POSITIVITY TRACKING

Write down three new and specific things you are grateful for today:

*1.*

*2.*

*3.*

## PARKING LOT

Write your thoughts and emotions out of your head and body and onto the page. Let go.

# Daily Expression

## Week 4/Date: _____

### HIT LIST

Write down three top priorities of the day that will move
the ball on your goals:

1. _____

2. _____

3. _____

### HYDRATION

Check off one droplet for each 8 ounces water you
consume today.

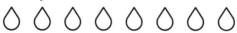

### MOVEMENT

What have I done today to move my body?

## MEALS

**BREAKFAST:** _____

☐ Protein: _____

☐ Fat: _____

☐ Fiber: _____

☐ Greens: _____


**LUNCH:** _____

☐ Protein: _____

☐ Fat: _____

☐ Fiber: _____

☐ Greens: _____


**DINNER:** _____

☐ Protein: _____

☐ Fat: _____

☐ Fiber: _____

☐ Greens: _____

TRACKING CHARTS

## POSITIVITY TRACKING

Write down three new and specific things you are grateful for today:

1.

2.

3.

## PARKING LOT

Write your thoughts and emotions out of your head and body and onto the page. Let go.

# Daily Expression

## Week 4/Date: _____

### HIT LIST

Write down three top priorities of the day that will move
the ball on your goals:

1. _____

2. _____

3. _____

### HYDRATION

Check off one droplet for each 8 ounces water you
consume today.

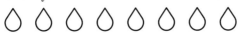

### MOVEMENT

What have I done today to move my body?

## MEALS

**BREAKFAST:** _____

☐ Protein: _____

☐ Fat: _____

☐ Fiber: _____

☐ Greens: _____


**LUNCH:** _____

☐ Protein: _____

☐ Fat: _____

☐ Fiber: _____

☐ Greens: _____


**DINNER:** _____

☐ Protein: _____

☐ Fat: _____

☐ Fiber: _____

☐ Greens: _____

## POSITIVITY TRACKING

Write down three new and specific things you are grateful for today:

1.

2.

3.

## PARKING LOT

Write your thoughts and emotions out of your head and body and onto the page. Let go.

# Daily Expression

**Week 4/Date:** _____

### HIT LIST

Write down three top priorities of the day that will move the ball on your goals:

*1.* _____

*2.* _____

*3.* _____

### HYDRATION

Check off one droplet for each 8 ounces water you consume today.

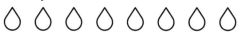

### MOVEMENT

What have I done today to move my body?

# MEALS

**BREAKFAST:** _____

☐ Protein: _____

☐ Fat: _____

☐ Fiber: _____

☐ Greens: _____


**LUNCH:** _____

☐ Protein: _____

☐ Fat: _____

☐ Fiber: _____

☐ Greens: _____


**DINNER:** _____

☐ Protein: _____

☐ Fat: _____

☐ Fiber: _____

☐ Greens: _____

TRACKING CHARTS

Write down three new and specific things you are grateful for today:

*1.*

*2.*

*3.*

Write your thoughts and emotions out of your head and body and onto the page. Let go.

BODY LOVE A JOURNAL

# Daily Expression

## Week 4/Date: _____

### HIT LIST

Write down three top priorities of the day that will move the ball on your goals:

*1.* _____

*2.* _____

*3.* _____

### HYDRATION

Check off one droplet for each 8 ounces water you consume today.

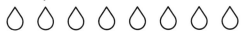

### MOVEMENT

What have I done today to move my body?

## MEALS

**BREAKFAST:** _____

☐ Protein: _____

☐ Fat: _____

☐ Fiber: _____

☐ Greens: _____


**LUNCH:** _____

☐ Protein: _____

☐ Fat: _____

☐ Fiber: _____

☐ Greens: _____


**DINNER:** _____

☐ Protein: _____

☐ Fat: _____

☐ Fiber: _____

☐ Greens: _____

## POSITIVITY TRACKING

Write down three new and specific things you are grateful for today:

1.

2.

3.

## PARKING LOT

Write your thoughts and emotions out of your head and body and onto the page. Let go.

# Daily Expression

## Week 4/Date: _____

### HIT LIST

Write down three top priorities of the day that will move the ball on your goals:

1. _____

2. _____

3. _____

### HYDRATION

Check off one droplet for each 8 ounces water you consume today.

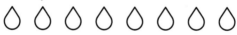

### MOVEMENT

What have I done today to move my body?

## MEALS

**BREAKFAST:** _____

☐ Protein: _____

☐ Fat: _____

☐ Fiber: _____

☐ Greens: _____


**LUNCH:** _____

☐ Protein: _____

☐ Fat: _____

☐ Fiber: _____

☐ Greens: _____


**DINNER:** _____

☐ Protein: _____

☐ Fat: _____

☐ Fiber: _____

☐ Greens: _____

TRACKING CHARTS

## POSITIVITY TRACKING

Write down three new and specific things you are grateful for today:

*1.*

*2.*

*3.*

## PARKING LOT

Write your thoughts and emotions out of your head and body and onto the page. Let go.

# Monthly Manifestation

**Month:** _____

### GO IN

Identify self-limiting beliefs and emotional patterns holding you back.

### LET GO

Take a moment to forgive yourself, release resentment, and erase regrets. It's time to let go of these beliefs and move forward.

## MANIFEST MAGIC

With nothing holding you back, visualize what your life would look like in a month, a year, five years, and ten years from now and write it down, being as specific as possible.

## MONTHLY SMART GOALS

Using the SMART goals framework on page 41, be specific about the repeatable and actionable steps you plan to take this month.

1. _____

2. _____

3. _____

# Weekly Planning

**Week 5:** _____

## SMOOTHIE INSPO

Write down three fun smoothie ideas for the next week:

1. _____

2. _____

3. _____

## #FAB4SMOOTHIE GROCERY LIST

☐ Liquid _____

    ☐ Nut Milk _____

    ☐ _____

☐ Protein _____

    ☐ Vanilla _____

    ☐ Chocolate _____

    ☐ _____

- ☐ Fat _____
  - ☐     Avocado _____
  - ☐     Nut Butter _____
  - ☐     Coconut _____
  - ☐     Healthy Oils _____
  - ☐     _____
- ☐ Fiber _____
  - ☐     Chia _____
  - ☐     Flax _____
  - ☐     Fiber Powders (acacia, psyllium husk) _____
- ☐ Greens _____
  - ☐     Fresh _____
  - ☐     Frozen _____
- ☐ Fruit _____
  - ☐     Fresh _____
    - ☐     Berries _____
    - ☐     Citrus _____
    - ☐     Tropical _____
  - ☐     Frozen _____
    - ☐     Berries _____

## WEEKLY MEAL PREP

Write down three great meal ideas for the next week:

1. _____

2. _____

3. _____

Which bulk protein do you want to use for your lunches?

_____

## FAB FOUR GROCERY LIST

☐ Protein

  ☐ _____

  ☐ _____

  ☐ _____

☐ Fat

  ☐ Cooking Oils

  ☐ Dressing

  ☐ Dip

☐ Nonstarchy Fiber-Rich Vegetables

    ☐ _____

    ☐ _____

    ☐ _____

    ☐ _____

☐ Greens

    ☐ Salad Greens _____

    ☐ Herbs _____

☐ Starch (one per week of savory and sweet)

    ☐ Savory _____

    ☐ Sweet _____

## ANCHOR APPOINTMENTS

**MONDAY**

**TUESDAY**

**WEDNESDAY**

**THURSDAY**

**FRIDAY**

**SATURDAY**

**SUNDAY**

# Daily Expression

**Week 5/Date:** _____

### HIT LIST

Write down three top priorities of the day that will move the ball on your goals:

*1.* _____

*2.* _____

*3.* _____

### HYDRATION

Check off one droplet for each 8 ounces water you consume today.

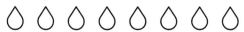

### MOVEMENT

What have I done today to move my body?

## MEALS

**BREAKFAST:** _____

- ☐ Protein: _____
- ☐ Fat: _____
- ☐ Fiber: _____
- ☐ Greens: _____

**LUNCH:** _____

- ☐ Protein: _____
- ☐ Fat: _____
- ☐ Fiber: _____
- ☐ Greens: _____

**DINNER:** _____

- ☐ Protein: _____
- ☐ Fat: _____
- ☐ Fiber: _____
- ☐ Greens: _____

## POSITIVITY TRACKING

Write down three new and specific things you are grateful for today:

*1.*

*2.*

*3.*

## PARKING LOT

Write your thoughts and emotions out of your head and body and onto the page. Let go.

# Daily Expression

**Week 5/Date:** _____

## HIT LIST

Write down three top priorities of the day that will move the ball on your goals:

1. _____

2. _____

3. _____

## HYDRATION

Check off one droplet for each 8 ounces water you consume today.

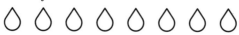

## MOVEMENT

What have I done today to move my body?

## MEALS

**BREAKFAST:** _____

☐ Protein: _____

☐ Fat: _____

☐ Fiber: _____

☐ Greens: _____


**LUNCH:** _____

☐ Protein: _____

☐ Fat: _____

☐ Fiber: _____

☐ Greens: _____


**DINNER:** _____

☐ Protein: _____

☐ Fat: _____

☐ Fiber: _____

☐ Greens: _____

TRACKING CHARTS

## POSITIVITY TRACKING

Write down three new and specific things you are grateful for today:

1.

2.

3.

## PARKING LOT

Write your thoughts and emotions out of your head and body and onto the page. Let go.

# Daily Expression

## Week 5/Date: _____

### HIT LIST

Write down three top priorities of the day that will move the ball on your goals:

*1.* _____

*2.* _____

*3.* _____

### HYDRATION

Check off one droplet for each 8 ounces water you consume today.

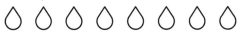

### MOVEMENT

What have I done today to move my body?

## MEALS

**BREAKFAST:** _____

☐ Protein: _____

☐ Fat: _____

☐ Fiber: _____

☐ Greens: _____


**LUNCH:** _____

☐ Protein: _____

☐ Fat: _____

☐ Fiber: _____

☐ Greens: _____


**DINNER:** _____

☐ Protein: _____

☐ Fat: _____

☐ Fiber: _____

☐ Greens: _____

## POSITIVITY TRACKING

Write down three new and specific things you are grateful for today:

1.

2.

3.

## PARKING LOT

Write your thoughts and emotions out of your head and body and onto the page. Let go.

# Daily Expression

## Week 5/Date: _____

### HIT LIST

Write down three top priorities of the day that will move
the ball on your goals:

1. _____

2. _____

3. _____

### HYDRATION

Check off one droplet for each 8 ounces water you
consume today.

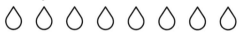

### MOVEMENT

What have I done today to move my body?

# MEALS

**BREAKFAST:** _____

☐ Protein: _____

☐ Fat: _____

☐ Fiber: _____

☐ Greens: _____


**LUNCH:** _____

☐ Protein: _____

☐ Fat: _____

☐ Fiber: _____

☐ Greens: _____


**DINNER:** _____

☐ Protein: _____

☐ Fat: _____

☐ Fiber: _____

☐ Greens: _____

TRACKING CHARTS

Write down three new and specific things you are grateful for today:

*1.*

*2.*

*3.*

## PARKING LOT

Write your thoughts and emotions out of your head and body and onto the page. Let go.

# Daily Expression

**Week 5/Date:** _____

## HIT LIST

Write down three top priorities of the day that will move
the ball on your goals:

1. _____

2. _____

3. _____

## HYDRATION

Check off one droplet for each 8 ounces water you
consume today.

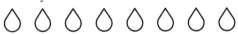

## MOVEMENT

What have I done today to move my body?

## MEALS

**BREAKFAST:** _____

☐ Protein: _____

☐ Fat: _____

☐ Fiber: _____

☐ Greens: _____


**LUNCH:** _____

☐ Protein: _____

☐ Fat: _____

☐ Fiber: _____

☐ Greens: _____


**DINNER:** _____

☐ Protein: _____

☐ Fat: _____

☐ Fiber: _____

☐ Greens: _____

## POSITIVITY TRACKING

Write down three new and specific things you are grateful for today:

1.

2.

3.

## PARKING LOT

Write your thoughts and emotions out of your head and body and onto the page. Let go.

# Daily Expression

BODY LOVE A JOURNAL

### HIT LIST

Write down three top priorities of the day that will move the ball on your goals:

1. _____

2. _____

3. _____

### HYDRATION

Check off one droplet for each 8 ounces water you consume today.

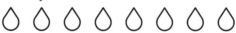

### MOVEMENT

What have I done today to move my body?

## MEALS

**BREAKFAST:** _____

- ☐ Protein: _____
- ☐ Fat: _____
- ☐ Fiber: _____
- ☐ Greens: _____


**LUNCH:** _____

- ☐ Protein: _____
- ☐ Fat: _____
- ☐ Fiber: _____
- ☐ Greens: _____


**DINNER:** _____

- ☐ Protein: _____
- ☐ Fat: _____
- ☐ Fiber: _____
- ☐ Greens: _____

## POSITIVITY TRACKING

Write down three new and specific things you are grateful for today:

*1.*

*2.*

*3.*

## PARKING LOT

Write your thoughts and emotions out of your head and body and onto the page. Let go.

# Daily Expression

**Week 5/Date:** _____

---

## HIT LIST

Write down three top priorities of the day that will move the ball on your goals:

1. _____

2. _____

3. _____

## HYDRATION

Check off one droplet for each 8 ounces water you consume today.

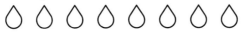

## MOVEMENT

What have I done today to move my body?

## MEALS

**BREAKFAST:** _____

☐ Protein: _____

☐ Fat: _____

☐ Fiber: _____

☐ Greens: _____


**LUNCH:** _____

☐ Protein: _____

☐ Fat: _____

☐ Fiber: _____

☐ Greens: _____


**DINNER:** _____

☐ Protein: _____

☐ Fat: _____

☐ Fiber: _____

☐ Greens: _____

BODY LOVE A JOURNAL

## POSITIVITY TRACKING

Write down three new and specific things you are grateful for today:

*1.*

*2.*

*3.*

## PARKING LOT

Write your thoughts and emotions out of your head and body and onto the page. Let go.

# Weekly Planning

**Week 6:** _____

## SMOOTHIE INSPO

Write down three fun smoothie ideas for the next week:

1. _____

2. _____

3. _____

## #FAB4SMOOTHIE GROCERY LIST

☐ Liquid _____

  ☐   Nut Milk _____

  ☐   _____

☐ Protein _____

  ☐   Vanilla _____

  ☐   Chocolate _____

  ☐   _____

☐ Fat _____

    ☐    Avocado _____

    ☐    Nut Butter _____

    ☐    Coconut _____

    ☐    Healthy Oils _____

    ☐    _____

☐ Fiber _____

    ☐    Chia _____

    ☐    Flax _____

    ☐    Fiber Powders (acacia, psyllium husk) _____

☐ Greens _____

    ☐    Fresh _____

    ☐    Frozen _____

☐ Fruit _____

    ☐    Fresh _____

        ☐    Berries _____

        ☐    Citrus _____

        ☐    Tropical _____

    ☐    Frozen _____

        ☐    Berries _____

Write down three great meal ideas for the next week:

1. _____

2. _____

3. _____

Which bulk protein do you want to use for your lunches?

_____

**FAB FOUR GROCERY LIST**

☐ Protein

    ☐ _____

    ☐ _____

    ☐ _____

☐ Fat

    ☐ Cooking Oils _____

    ☐ Dressing _____

    ☐ Dip _____

☐ Nonstarchy Fiber-Rich Vegetables

    ☐ _____

    ☐ _____

    ☐ _____

    ☐ _____

☐ Greens

    ☐ Salad Greens _____

    ☐ Herbs _____

☐ Starch (one per week of savory and sweet)

    ☐ Savory _____

    ☐ Sweet _____

## ANCHOR APPOINTMENTS

**MONDAY**

**TUESDAY**

**WEDNESDAY**

**THURSDAY**

**FRIDAY**

**SATURDAY**

**SUNDAY**

# Daily Expression

**Week 6/Date:** _____

## HIT LIST

Write down three top priorities of the day that will move the ball on your goals:

*1.* _____

*2.* _____

*3.* _____

## HYDRATION

Check off one droplet for each 8 ounces water you consume today.

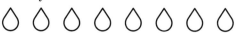

## MOVEMENT

What have I done today to move my body?

# MEALS

**BREAKFAST:** _____

☐ Protein: _____

☐ Fat: _____

☐ Fiber: _____

☐ Greens: _____


**LUNCH:** _____

☐ Protein: _____

☐ Fat: _____

☐ Fiber: _____

☐ Greens: _____


**DINNER:** _____

☐ Protein: _____

☐ Fat: _____

☐ Fiber: _____

☐ Greens: _____

TRACKING CHARTS

Write down three new and specific things you are grateful for today:

*1.*

*2.*

*3.*

Write your thoughts and emotions out of your head and body and onto the page. Let go.

BODY LOVE A JOURNAL

# Daily Expression

**Week 6/Date:** _____

## HIT LIST

Write down three top priorities of the day that will move the ball on your goals:

1. _____

2. _____

3. _____

## HYDRATION

Check off one droplet for each 8 ounces water you consume today.

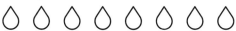

## MOVEMENT

What have I done today to move my body?

**BREAKFAST:** _____

☐ Protein: _____

☐ Fat: _____

☐ Fiber: _____

☐ Greens: _____

**LUNCH:** _____

☐ Protein: _____

☐ Fat: _____

☐ Fiber: _____

☐ Greens: _____

**DINNER:** _____

☐ Protein: _____

☐ Fat: _____

☐ Fiber: _____

☐ Greens: _____

## POSITIVITY TRACKING

Write down three new and specific things you are grateful for today:

*1.*

*2.*

*3.*

## PARKING LOT

Write your thoughts and emotions out of your head and body and onto the page. Let go.

# Daily Expression

## Week 6/Date: _____

### HIT LIST

Write down three top priorities of the day that will move the ball on your goals:

1. _____

2. _____

3. _____

### HYDRATION

Check off one droplet for each 8 ounces water you consume today.

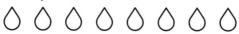

### MOVEMENT

What have I done today to move my body?

## MEALS

**BREAKFAST:** _____

- ☐ Protein: _____
- ☐ Fat: _____
- ☐ Fiber: _____
- ☐ Greens: _____

**LUNCH:** _____

- ☐ Protein: _____
- ☐ Fat: _____
- ☐ Fiber: _____
- ☐ Greens: _____

**DINNER:** _____

- ☐ Protein: _____
- ☐ Fat: _____
- ☐ Fiber: _____
- ☐ Greens: _____

TRACKING CHARTS

197

## POSITIVITY TRACKING

Write down three new and specific things you are grateful for today:

*1.*

*2.*

*3.*

## PARKING LOT

Write your thoughts and emotions out of your head and body and onto the page. Let go.

# Daily Expression

**Week 6/Date:** _____

### HIT LIST

Write down three top priorities of the day that will move the ball on your goals:

1. _____

2. _____

3. _____

### HYDRATION

Check off one droplet for each 8 ounces water you consume today.

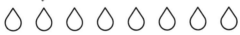

### MOVEMENT

What have I done today to move my body?

## MEALS

**BREAKFAST:** _____

- ☐  Protein: _____
- ☐  Fat: _____
- ☐  Fiber: _____
- ☐  Greens: _____


**LUNCH:** _____

- ☐  Protein: _____
- ☐  Fat: _____
- ☐  Fiber: _____
- ☐  Greens: _____


**DINNER:** _____

- ☐  Protein: _____
- ☐  Fat: _____
- ☐  Fiber: _____
- ☐  Greens: _____

## POSITIVITY TRACKING

Write down three new and specific things you are grateful for today:

1.

2.

3.

## PARKING LOT

Write your thoughts and emotions out of your head and body and onto the page. Let go.

# Daily Expression

## Week 6/Date: _____

### HIT LIST

Write down three top priorities of the day that will move
the ball on your goals:

1. _____

2. _____

3. _____

### HYDRATION

Check off one droplet for each 8 ounces water you
consume today.

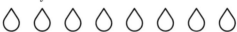

### MOVEMENT

What have I done today to move my body?

# MEALS

**BREAKFAST:** _____

- ☐ Protein: _____
- ☐ Fat: _____
- ☐ Fiber: _____
- ☐ Greens: _____

**LUNCH:** _____

- ☐ Protein: _____
- ☐ Fat: _____
- ☐ Fiber: _____
- ☐ Greens: _____

**DINNER:** _____

- ☐ Protein: _____
- ☐ Fat: _____
- ☐ Fiber: _____
- ☐ Greens: _____

Write down three new and specific things you are grateful for today:

*1.*

*2.*

*3.*

## PARKING LOT

Write your thoughts and emotions out of your head and body and onto the page. Let go.

# Daily Expression

**Week 6/Date:** _____

### HIT LIST

Write down three top priorities of the day that will move the ball on your goals:

*1.* _____

*2.* _____

*3.* _____

### HYDRATION

Check off one droplet for each 8 ounces water you consume today.

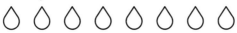

### MOVEMENT

What have I done today to move my body?

## MEALS

**BREAKFAST:** _____

☐  Protein: _____

☐  Fat: _____

☐  Fiber: _____

☐  Greens: _____


**LUNCH:** _____

☐  Protein: _____

☐  Fat: _____

☐  Fiber: _____

☐  Greens: _____


**DINNER:** _____

☐  Protein: _____

☐  Fat: _____

☐  Fiber: _____

☐  Greens: _____

## POSITIVITY TRACKING

Write down three new and specific things you are grateful for today:

1.

2.

3.

## PARKING LOT

Write your thoughts and emotions out of your head and body and onto the page. Let go.

# Daily Expression

## Week 6/Date: _____

### HIT LIST

Write down three top priorities of the day that will move the ball on your goals:

1. _____

2. _____

3. _____

### HYDRATION

Check off one droplet for each 8 ounces water you consume today.

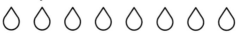

### MOVEMENT

What have I done today to move my body?

# MEALS

**BREAKFAST:** _____

☐ Protein: _____

☐ Fat: _____

☐ Fiber: _____

☐ Greens: _____


**LUNCH:** _____

☐ Protein: _____

☐ Fat: _____

☐ Fiber: _____

☐ Greens: _____


**DINNER:** _____

☐ Protein: _____

☐ Fat: _____

☐ Fiber: _____

☐ Greens: _____

## POSITIVITY TRACKING

Write down three new and specific things you are grateful for today:

*1.*

*2.*

*3.*

## PARKING LOT

Write your thoughts and emotions out of your head and body and onto the page. Let go.

# Weekly Planning

**Week 7:** _____

## SMOOTHIE INSPO

Write down three fun smoothie ideas for the next week:

1. _____

2. _____

3. _____

## #FAB4SMOOTHIE GROCERY LIST

☐ Liquid _____

   ☐   Nut Milk _____

   ☐   _____

☐ Protein _____

   ☐   Vanilla _____

   ☐   Chocolate _____

   ☐   _____

- ☐ Fat _____
  - ☐ Avocado _____
  - ☐ Nut Butter _____
  - ☐ Coconut _____
  - ☐ Healthy Oils _____
  - ☐ _____

- ☐ Fiber _____
  - ☐ Chia _____
  - ☐ Flax _____
  - ☐ Fiber Powders (acacia, psyllium husk) _____

- ☐ Greens _____
  - ☐ Fresh _____
  - ☐ Frozen _____

- ☐ Fruit _____
  - ☐ Fresh _____
    - ☐ Berries _____
    - ☐ Citrus _____
    - ☐ Tropical _____
  - ☐ Frozen _____
    - ☐ Berries _____

## WEEKLY MEAL PREP

Write down three great meal ideas for the next week:

*1.* _____

*2.* _____

*3.* _____

Which bulk protein do you want to use for your lunches?

_____

## FAB FOUR GROCERY LIST

☐ Protein

   ☐ _____

   ☐ _____

   ☐ _____

☐ Fat

   ☐ Cooking Oils _____

   ☐ Dressing _____

   ☐ Dip _____

☐ Nonstarchy Fiber-Rich Vegetables

   ☐ _____

   ☐ _____

   ☐ _____

   ☐ _____

☐ Greens

   ☐ Salad Greens _____

   ☐ Herbs _____

☐ Starch (one per week of savory and sweet)

   ☐ Savory _____

   ☐ Sweet _____

## ANCHOR APPOINTMENTS

**MONDAY**

**TUESDAY**

**WEDNESDAY**

**THURSDAY**

**FRIDAY**

**SATURDAY**

**SUNDAY**

# Daily Expression

**Week 7/Date:** _____

---

### HIT LIST

Write down three top priorities of the day that will move the ball on your goals:

1. _____

2. _____

3. _____

---

### HYDRATION

Check off one droplet for each 8 ounces water you consume today.

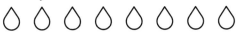

---

### MOVEMENT

What have I done today to move my body?

## MEALS

**BREAKFAST:** _____

- ☐ Protein: _____
- ☐ Fat: _____
- ☐ Fiber: _____
- ☐ Greens: _____

**LUNCH:** _____

- ☐ Protein: _____
- ☐ Fat: _____
- ☐ Fiber: _____
- ☐ Greens: _____

**DINNER:** _____

- ☐ Protein: _____
- ☐ Fat: _____
- ☐ Fiber: _____
- ☐ Greens: _____

## POSITIVITY TRACKING

Write down three new and specific things you are grateful for today:

1.

2.

3.

## PARKING LOT

Write your thoughts and emotions out of your head and body and onto the page. Let go.

# Daily Expression

## Week 7/Date: _____

**HIT LIST**

Write down three top priorities of the day that will move
the ball on your goals:

*1.* _____

*2.* _____

*3.* _____

**HYDRATION**

Check off one droplet for each 8 ounces water you
consume today.

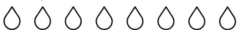

**MOVEMENT**

What have I done today to move my body?

# MEALS

**BREAKFAST:** _____

☐ Protein: _____

☐ Fat: _____

☐ Fiber: _____

☐ Greens: _____


**LUNCH:** _____

☐ Protein: _____

☐ Fat: _____

☐ Fiber: _____

☐ Greens: _____


**DINNER:** _____

☐ Protein: _____

☐ Fat: _____

☐ Fiber: _____

☐ Greens: _____

TRACKING CHARTS

## POSITIVITY TRACKING

Write down three new and specific things you are grateful for today:

*1.*

*2.*

*3.*

## PARKING LOT

Write your thoughts and emotions out of your head and body and onto the page. Let go.

# Daily Expression

## HIT LIST

Write down three top priorities of the day that will move
the ball on your goals:

1. _____

2. _____

3. _____

## HYDRATION

Check off one droplet for each 8 ounces water you
consume today.

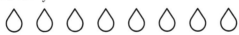

## MOVEMENT

What have I done today to move my body?

## MEALS

**BREAKFAST:** _____

- ☐ Protein: _____
- ☐ Fat: _____
- ☐ Fiber: _____
- ☐ Greens: _____

**LUNCH:** _____

- ☐ Protein: _____
- ☐ Fat: _____
- ☐ Fiber: _____
- ☐ Greens: _____

**DINNER:** _____

- ☐ Protein: _____
- ☐ Fat: _____
- ☐ Fiber: _____
- ☐ Greens: _____

## POSITIVITY TRACKING

Write down three new and specific things you are grateful for today:

*1.*

*2.*

*3.*

## PARKING LOT

Write your thoughts and emotions out of your head and body and onto the page. Let go.

# Daily Expression

**Week 7/Date:** _____

## HIT LIST

Write down three top priorities of the day that will move
the ball on your goals:

1. _____

2. _____

3. _____

## HYDRATION

Check off one droplet for each 8 ounces water you
consume today.

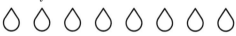

## MOVEMENT

What have I done today to move my body?

## MEALS

**BREAKFAST:** _____

- ☐ Protein: _____
- ☐ Fat: _____
- ☐ Fiber: _____
- ☐ Greens: _____

**LUNCH:** _____

- ☐ Protein: _____
- ☐ Fat: _____
- ☐ Fiber: _____
- ☐ Greens: _____

**DINNER:** _____

- ☐ Protein: _____
- ☐ Fat: _____
- ☐ Fiber: _____
- ☐ Greens: _____

## POSITIVITY TRACKING

Write down three new and specific things you are grateful for today:

*1.*

*2.*

*3.*

## PARKING LOT

Write your thoughts and emotions out of your head and body and onto the page. Let go.

# Daily Expression

**Week 7/Date:** _____

## HIT LIST

Write down three top priorities of the day that will move the ball on your goals:

1. _____

2. _____

3. _____

## HYDRATION

Check off one droplet for each 8 ounces water you consume today.

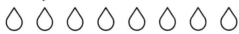

## MOVEMENT

What have I done today to move my body?

## MEALS

**BREAKFAST:** _____

- ☐ Protein: _____

- ☐ Fat: _____

- ☐ Fiber: _____

- ☐ Greens: _____


**LUNCH:** _____

- ☐ Protein: _____

- ☐ Fat: _____

- ☐ Fiber: _____

- ☐ Greens: _____


**DINNER:** _____

- ☐ Protein: _____

- ☐ Fat: _____

- ☐ Fiber: _____

- ☐ Greens: _____

Write down three new and specific things you are grateful for today:

1.

2.

3.

Write your thoughts and emotions out of your head and body and onto the page. Let go.

# Daily Expression

## Week 7/Date: _____

### HIT LIST

Write down three top priorities of the day that will move
the ball on your goals:

1. _____

2. _____

3. _____

### HYDRATION

Check off one droplet for each 8 ounces water you
consume today.

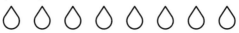

### MOVEMENT

What have I done today to move my body?

# MEALS

**BREAKFAST:** _____

☐  Protein: _____

☐  Fat: _____

☐  Fiber: _____

☐  Greens: _____


**LUNCH:** _____

☐  Protein: _____

☐  Fat: _____

☐  Fiber: _____

☐  Greens: _____


**DINNER:** _____

☐  Protein: _____

☐  Fat: _____

☐  Fiber: _____

☐  Greens: _____

## POSITIVITY TRACKING

Write down three new and specific things you are grateful for today:

*1.*

*2.*

*3.*

## PARKING LOT

Write your thoughts and emotions out of your head and body and onto the page. Let go.

# Daily Expression

**Week 7/Date:** _____

## HIT LIST

Write down three top priorities of the day that will move the ball on your goals:

*1.* _____

*2.* _____

*3.* _____

## HYDRATION

Check off one droplet for each 8 ounces water you consume today.

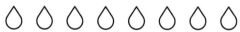

## MOVEMENT

What have I done today to move my body?

## MEALS

**BREAKFAST:** _____

☐  Protein: _____

☐  Fat: _____

☐  Fiber: _____

☐  Greens: _____


**LUNCH:** _____

☐  Protein: _____

☐  Fat: _____

☐  Fiber: _____

☐  Greens: _____


**DINNER:** _____

☐  Protein: _____

☐  Fat: _____

☐  Fiber: _____

☐  Greens: _____

BODY LOVE A JOURNAL

## POSITIVITY TRACKING

Write down three new and specific things you are grateful for today:

1.

2.

3.

## PARKING LOT

Write your thoughts and emotions out of your head and body and onto the page. Let go.

# Weekly Planning

**Week 8:** _____

---

### SMOOTHIE INSPO

Write down three fun smoothie ideas for the next week:

*1.* _____

*2.* _____

*3.* _____

---

### #FAB4SMOOTHIE GROCERY LIST

☐ Liquid _____

   ☐   Nut Milk _____

   ☐   _____

☐ Protein _____

   ☐   Vanilla _____

   ☐   Chocolate _____

   ☐   _____

- ☐ Fat _____
  - ☐ Avocado _____
  - ☐ Nut Butter _____
  - ☐ Coconut _____
  - ☐ Healthy Oils _____
  - ☐ _____
- ☐ Fiber _____
  - ☐ Chia _____
  - ☐ Flax _____
  - ☐ Fiber Powders (acacia, psyllium husk) ___
- ☐ Greens _____
  - ☐ Fresh _____
  - ☐ Frozen _____
- ☐ Fruit _____
  - ☐ Fresh _____
    - ☐ Berries _____
    - ☐ Citrus _____
    - ☐ Tropical _____
  - ☐ Frozen _____
    - ☐ Berries _____

Write down three great meal ideas for the next week:

*1.* _____

*2.* _____

*3.* _____

Which bulk protein do you want to use for your lunches?

_____

**FAB FOUR GROCERY LIST**

☐ Protein

    ☐ _____

    ☐ _____

    ☐ _____

☐ Fat

    ☐ Cooking Oils _____

    ☐ Dressing _____

    ☐ Dip _____

☐ Nonstarchy Fiber-Rich Vegetables

    ☐ _____

    ☐ _____

    ☐ _____

    ☐ _____

☐ Greens

    ☐ Salad Greens _____

    ☐ Herbs _____

☐ Starch (one per week of savory and sweet)

    ☐ Savory _____

    ☐ Sweet _____

## ANCHOR APPOINTMENTS

**MONDAY**

**TUESDAY**

**WEDNESDAY**

**THURSDAY**

**FRIDAY**

**SATURDAY**

**SUNDAY**

# Daily Expression

## Week 8/Date: _____

**HIT LIST**

Write down three top priorities of the day that will move the ball on your goals:

*1.* _____

*2.* _____

*3.* _____

**HYDRATION**

Check off one droplet for each 8 ounces water you consume today.

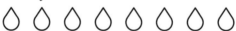

**MOVEMENT**

What have I done today to move my body?

## MEALS

**BREAKFAST:** _____

- ☐ Protein: _____
- ☐ Fat: _____
- ☐ Fiber: _____
- ☐ Greens: _____

**LUNCH:** _____

- ☐ Protein: _____
- ☐ Fat: _____
- ☐ Fiber: _____
- ☐ Greens: _____

**DINNER:** _____

- ☐ Protein: _____
- ☐ Fat: _____
- ☐ Fiber: _____
- ☐ Greens: _____

TRACKING CHARTS

## POSITIVITY TRACKING

Write down three new and specific things you are grateful for today:

1.

2.

3.

## PARKING LOT

Write your thoughts and emotions out of your head and body and onto the page. Let go.

BODY LOVE A JOURNAL

# Daily Expression

**Week 8/Date:** _____

## HIT LIST

Write down three top priorities of the day that will move the ball on your goals:

1. _____

2. _____

3. _____

## HYDRATION

Check off one droplet for each 8 ounces water you consume today.

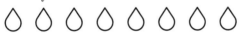

## MOVEMENT

What have I done today to move my body?

243

**BREAKFAST:** _____

☐ Protein: _____

☐ Fat: _____

☐ Fiber: _____

☐ Greens: _____


**LUNCH:** _____

☐ Protein: _____

☐ Fat: _____

☐ Fiber: _____

☐ Greens: _____


**DINNER:** _____

☐ Protein: _____

☐ Fat: _____

☐ Fiber: _____

☐ Greens: _____

BODY LOVE A JOURNAL

## POSITIVITY TRACKING

Write down three new and specific things you are grateful for today:

1.

2.

3.

## PARKING LOT

Write your thoughts and emotions out of your head and body and onto the page. Let go.

# Daily Expression

## Week 8/Date: _____

### HIT LIST

Write down three top priorities of the day that will move
the ball on your goals:

1. _____

2. _____

3. _____

### HYDRATION

Check off one droplet for each 8 ounces water you
consume today.

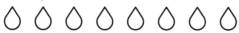

### MOVEMENT

What have I done today to move my body?

# MEALS

**BREAKFAST:** _____

☐ Protein: _____

☐ Fat: _____

☐ Fiber: _____

☐ Greens: _____


**LUNCH:** _____

☐ Protein: _____

☐ Fat: _____

☐ Fiber: _____

☐ Greens: _____


**DINNER:** _____

☐ Protein: _____

☐ Fat: _____

☐ Fiber: _____

☐ Greens: _____

TRACKING CHARTS

247

## POSITIVITY TRACKING

Write down three new and specific things you are grateful for today:

1.

2.

3.

## PARKING LOT

Write your thoughts and emotions out of your head and body and onto the page. Let go.

# Daily Expression

**Week 8/Date:** _____

### HIT LIST

Write down three top priorities of the day that will move the ball on your goals:

*1.* _____

*2.* _____

*3.* _____

### HYDRATION

Check off one droplet for each 8 ounces water you consume today.

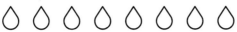

### MOVEMENT

What have I done today to move my body?

## MEALS

**BREAKFAST:** _____

☐ Protein: _____

☐ Fat: _____

☐ Fiber: _____

☐ Greens: _____


**LUNCH:** _____

☐ Protein: _____

☐ Fat: _____

☐ Fiber: _____

☐ Greens: _____


**DINNER:** _____

☐ Protein: _____

☐ Fat: _____

☐ Fiber: _____

☐ Greens: _____

## POSITIVITY TRACKING

Write down three new and specific things you are grateful for today:

1.


2.


3.


## PARKING LOT

Write your thoughts and emotions out of your head and body and onto the page. Let go.

# Daily Expression

## Week 8/Date: _____

### HIT LIST

Write down three top priorities of the day that will move
the ball on your goals:

1. _____

2. _____

3. _____

### HYDRATION

Check off one droplet for each 8 ounces water you
consume today.

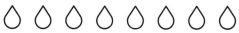

### MOVEMENT

What have I done today to move my body?

# MEALS

**BREAKFAST:** _____

- ☐ Protein: _____
- ☐ Fat: _____
- ☐ Fiber: _____
- ☐ Greens: _____


**LUNCH:** _____

- ☐ Protein: _____
- ☐ Fat: _____
- ☐ Fiber: _____
- ☐ Greens: _____


**DINNER:** _____

- ☐ Protein: _____
- ☐ Fat: _____
- ☐ Fiber: _____
- ☐ Greens: _____

TRACKING CHARTS

## POSITIVITY TRACKING

Write down three new and specific things you are grateful for today:

*1.*

*2.*

*3.*

## PARKING LOT

Write your thoughts and emotions out of your head and body and onto the page. Let go.

# Daily Expression

**Week 8/Date:** _____

### HIT LIST

Write down three top priorities of the day that will move the ball on your goals:

*1.* _____

*2.* _____

*3.* _____

### HYDRATION

Check off one droplet for each 8 ounces water you consume today.

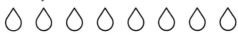

### MOVEMENT

What have I done today to move my body?

## MEALS

**BREAKFAST:** _____

☐ Protein: _____

☐ Fat: _____

☐ Fiber: _____

☐ Greens: _____

**LUNCH:** _____

☐ Protein: _____

☐ Fat: _____

☐ Fiber: _____

☐ Greens: _____

**DINNER:** _____

☐ Protein: _____

☐ Fat: _____

☐ Fiber: _____

☐ Greens: _____

## POSITIVITY TRACKING

Write down three new and specific things you are grateful for today:

*1.*

*2.*

*3.*

## PARKING LOT

Write your thoughts and emotions out of your head and body and onto the page. Let go.

# Daily Expression

**Week 8/Date:** _____

### HIT LIST

Write down three top priorities of the day that will move the ball on your goals:

*1.* _____

*2.* _____

*3.* _____

### HYDRATION

Check off one droplet for each 8 ounces water you consume today.

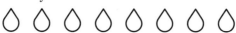

### MOVEMENT

What have I done today to move my body?

# MEALS

**BREAKFAST:** _____

☐ Protein: _____

☐ Fat: _____

☐ Fiber: _____

☐ Greens: _____


**LUNCH:** _____

☐ Protein: _____

☐ Fat: _____

☐ Fiber: _____

☐ Greens: _____


**DINNER:** _____

☐ Protein: _____

☐ Fat: _____

☐ Fiber: _____

☐ Greens: _____

TRACKING CHARTS

259

## POSITIVITY TRACKING

Write down three new and specific things you are grateful for today:

*1.*

*2.*

*3.*

## PARKING LOT

Write your thoughts and emotions out of your head and body and onto the page. Let go.

# Monthly Manifestation

**Month:** _____

## GO IN

Identify self-limiting beliefs and emotional patterns
holding you back.

## LET GO

Take a moment to forgive yourself, release resentment,
and erase regrets. It's time to let go of these beliefs and
move forward.

## MANIFEST MAGIC

With nothing holding you back, visualize what your life would look like in a month, a year, five years, and ten years from now and write it down, being as specific as possible.

## MONTHLY SMART GOALS

Using the SMART goals framework on page 41, be specific about the repeatable and actionable steps you plan to take this month.

1. _____

2. _____

3. _____

# Weekly Planning

**Week 9:** _____

## SMOOTHIE INSPO

Write down three fun smoothie ideas for the next week:

1. _____

2. _____

3. _____

## #FAB4SMOOTHIE GROCERY LIST

☐ Liquid _____

   ☐ Nut Milk _____

   ☐ _____

☐ Protein _____

   ☐ Vanilla _____

   ☐ Chocolate _____

   ☐ _____

☐ Fat _____

    ☐ Avocado _____

    ☐ Nut Butter _____

    ☐ Coconut _____

    ☐ Healthy Oils _____

    ☐ _____

☐ Fiber _____

    ☐ Chia _____

    ☐ Flax _____

    ☐ Fiber Powders (acacia, psyllium husk) _____

☐ Greens _____

    ☐ Fresh _____

    ☐ Frozen _____

☐ Fruit _____

    ☐ Fresh _____

        ☐ Berries _____

        ☐ Citrus _____

        ☐ Tropical _____

    ☐ Frozen _____

        ☐ Berries _____

## WEEKLY MEAL PREP

Write down three great meal ideas for the next week:

1. _____

2. _____

3. _____

Which bulk protein do you want to use for your lunches?

_____

## FAB FOUR GROCERY LIST

☐ Protein

   ☐ _____

   ☐ _____

   ☐ _____

☐ Fat

   ☐ Cooking Oils

   ☐ Dressing

   ☐ Dip

☐ Nonstarchy Fiber-Rich Vegetables

   ☐ _____

   ☐ _____

   ☐ _____

   ☐ _____

☐ Greens

   ☐ Salad Greens _____

   ☐ Herbs _____

☐ Starch (one per week of savory and sweet)

   ☐ Savory _____

   ☐ Sweet _____

## ANCHOR APPOINTMENTS

**MONDAY**

**TUESDAY**

**WEDNESDAY**

**THURSDAY**

**FRIDAY**

**SATURDAY**

**SUNDAY**

# Daily Expression

**Week 9/Date:** _____

## HIT LIST

Write down three top priorities of the day that will move the ball on your goals:

*1.* _____

*2.* _____

*3.* _____

## HYDRATION

Check off one droplet for each 8 ounces water you consume today.

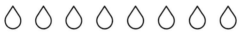

## MOVEMENT

What have I done today to move my body?

**BREAKFAST:** _____

☐ Protein: _____

☐ Fat: _____

☐ Fiber: _____

☐ Greens: _____


**LUNCH:** _____

☐ Protein: _____

☐ Fat: _____

☐ Fiber: _____

☐ Greens: _____


**DINNER:** _____

☐ Protein: _____

☐ Fat: _____

☐ Fiber: _____

☐ Greens: _____

## POSITIVITY TRACKING

Write down three new and specific things you are grateful for today:

*1.*

*2.*

*3.*

## PARKING LOT

Write your thoughts and emotions out of your head and body and onto the page. Let go.

# Daily Expression

## Week 9/Date: _____

### HIT LIST

Write down three top priorities of the day that will move the ball on your goals:

1. _____

2. _____

3. _____

### HYDRATION

Check off one droplet for each 8 ounces water you consume today.

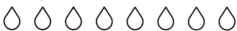

### MOVEMENT

What have I done today to move my body?

# MEALS

**BREAKFAST:** _____

☐ Protein: _____

☐ Fat: _____

☐ Fiber: _____

☐ Greens: _____


**LUNCH:** _____

☐ Protein: _____

☐ Fat: _____

☐ Fiber: _____

☐ Greens: _____


**DINNER:** _____

☐ Protein: _____

☐ Fat: _____

☐ Fiber: _____

☐ Greens: _____

TRACKING CHARTS

271

## POSITIVITY TRACKING

Write down three new and specific things you are grateful for today:

1.

2.

3.

## PARKING LOT

Write your thoughts and emotions out of your head and body and onto the page. Let go.

# Daily Expression

**Week 9/Date:** _____

## HIT LIST

Write down three top priorities of the day that will move
the ball on your goals:

1. _____

2. _____

3. _____

## HYDRATION

Check off one droplet for each 8 ounces water you
consume today.

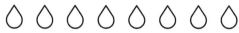

## MOVEMENT

What have I done today to move my body?

## MEALS

**BREAKFAST:** _____

☐ Protein: _____

☐ Fat: _____

☐ Fiber: _____

☐ Greens: _____


**LUNCH:** _____

☐ Protein: _____

☐ Fat: _____

☐ Fiber: _____

☐ Greens: _____


**DINNER:** _____

☐ Protein: _____

☐ Fat: _____

☐ Fiber: _____

☐ Greens: _____

## POSITIVITY TRACKING

Write down three new and specific things you are grateful for today:

*1.*

*2.*

*3.*

## PARKING LOT

Write your thoughts and emotions out of your head and body and onto the page. Let go.

# Daily Expression

## Week 9/Date: _____

### HIT LIST

Write down three top priorities of the day that will move
the ball on your goals:

1. _____

2. _____

3. _____

### HYDRATION

Check off one droplet for each 8 ounces water you
consume today.

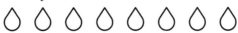

### MOVEMENT

What have I done today to move my body?

276

## MEALS

**BREAKFAST:** _____

☐ Protein: _____

☐ Fat: _____

☐ Fiber: _____

☐ Greens: _____


**LUNCH:** _____

☐ Protein: _____

☐ Fat: _____

☐ Fiber: _____

☐ Greens: _____


**DINNER:** _____

☐ Protein: _____

☐ Fat: _____

☐ Fiber: _____

☐ Greens: _____

TRACKING CHARTS

## POSITIVITY TRACKING

Write down three new and specific things you are grateful for today:

*1.*

*2.*

*3.*

## PARKING LOT

Write your thoughts and emotions out of your head and body and onto the page. Let go.

# Daily Expression

**Week 9/Date:** _____

## HIT LIST

Write down three top priorities of the day that will move
the ball on your goals:

*1.* _____

*2.* _____

*3.* _____

## HYDRATION

Check off one droplet for each 8 ounces water you
consume today.

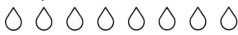

## MOVEMENT

What have I done today to move my body?

## MEALS

**BREAKFAST:** _____

☐ Protein: _____

☐ Fat: _____

☐ Fiber: _____

☐ Greens: _____


**LUNCH:** _____

☐ Protein: _____

☐ Fat: _____

☐ Fiber: _____

☐ Greens: _____


**DINNER:** _____

☐ Protein: _____

☐ Fat: _____

☐ Fiber: _____

☐ Greens: _____

## POSITIVITY TRACKING

Write down three new and specific things you are grateful for today:

*1.*

*2.*

*3.*

## PARKING LOT

Write your thoughts and emotions out of your head and body and onto the page. Let go.

# Daily Expression

## Week 9/Date: _____

### HIT LIST

Write down three top priorities of the day that will move the ball on your goals:

1. _____

2. _____

3. _____

### HYDRATION

Check off one droplet for each 8 ounces water you consume today.

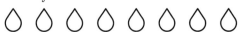

### MOVEMENT

What have I done today to move my body?

# MEALS

**BREAKFAST:** _____

☐ Protein: _____

☐ Fat: _____

☐ Fiber: _____

☐ Greens: _____


**LUNCH:** _____

☐ Protein: _____

☐ Fat: _____

☐ Fiber: _____

☐ Greens: _____


**DINNER:** _____

☐ Protein: _____

☐ Fat: _____

☐ Fiber: _____

☐ Greens: _____

## POSITIVITY TRACKING

Write down three new and specific things you are grateful for today:

1.

2.

3.

## PARKING LOT

Write your thoughts and emotions out of your head and body and onto the page. Let go.

# Daily Expression

**Week 9/Date:** _____

## HIT LIST

Write down three top priorities of the day that will move the ball on your goals:

1. _____

2. _____

3. _____

## HYDRATION

Check off one droplet for each 8 ounces water you consume today.

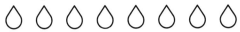

## MOVEMENT

What have I done today to move my body?

TRACKING CHARTS

**BREAKFAST:** _____

☐ Protein: _____

☐ Fat: _____

☐ Fiber: _____

☐ Greens: _____


**LUNCH:** _____

☐ Protein: _____

☐ Fat: _____

☐ Fiber: _____

☐ Greens: _____


**DINNER:** _____

☐ Protein: _____

☐ Fat: _____

☐ Fiber: _____

☐ Greens: _____

## POSITIVITY TRACKING

Write down three new and specific things you are grateful for today:

1.

2.

3.

## PARKING LOT

Write your thoughts and emotions out of your head and body and onto the page. Let go.

# Weekly Planning

---

**SMOOTHIE INSPO**

Write down three fun smoothie ideas for the next week:

1. _____

2. _____

3. _____

**#FAB4SMOOTHIE GROCERY LIST**

☐  Liquid _____

    ☐  Nut Milk _____

    ☐  _____

☐  Protein _____

    ☐  Vanilla _____

    ☐  Chocolate _____

    ☐  _____

- ☐ Fat _____
  - ☐    Avocado _____
  - ☐    Nut Butter _____
  - ☐    Coconut _____
  - ☐    Healthy Oils _____
  - ☐    _____
- ☐ Fiber _____
  - ☐    Chia _____
  - ☐    Flax _____
  - ☐    Fiber Powders (acacia, psyllium husk) _____
- ☐ Greens _____
  - ☐    Fresh _____
  - ☐    Frozen _____
- ☐ Fruit _____
  - ☐    Fresh _____
    - ☐    Berries _____
    - ☐    Citrus _____
    - ☐    Tropical _____
  - ☐    Frozen _____
    - ☐    Berries _____

Write down three great meal ideas for the next week:

1. _____

2. _____

3. _____

Which bulk protein do you want to use for your lunches?

_____

## FAB FOUR GROCERY LIST

☐ Protein

    ☐ _____

    ☐ _____

    ☐ _____

☐ Fat

    ☐ Cooking Oils _____

    ☐ Dressing _____

    ☐ Dip _____

☐ Nonstarchy Fiber-Rich Vegetables

   ☐ _____

   ☐ _____

   ☐ _____

   ☐ _____

☐ Greens

   ☐ Salad Greens

   ☐ Herbs

☐ Starch (one per week of savory and sweet)

   ☐ Savory

   ☐ Sweet

## ANCHOR APPOINTMENTS

**MONDAY**

**TUESDAY**

**WEDNESDAY**

**THURSDAY**

**FRIDAY**

**SATURDAY**

**SUNDAY**

# Daily Expression

**Week 10/Date:** _____

## HIT LIST

Write down three top priorities of the day that will move
the ball on your goals:

1. _____

2. _____

3. _____

## HYDRATION

Check off one droplet for each 8 ounces water you
consume today.

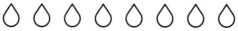

## MOVEMENT

What have I done today to move my body?

## MEALS

**BREAKFAST:** _____

☐  Protein: _____

☐  Fat: _____

☐  Fiber: _____

☐  Greens: _____


**LUNCH:** _____

☐  Protein: _____

☐  Fat: _____

☐  Fiber: _____

☐  Greens: _____


**DINNER:** _____

☐  Protein: _____

☐  Fat: _____

☐  Fiber: _____

☐  Greens: _____

Write down three new and specific things you are grateful for today:

*1.*

2.

*3.*

## PARKING LOT

Write your thoughts and emotions out of your head and body and onto the page. Let go.

# Daily Expression

**Week 10/Date: _____**

## HIT LIST

Write down three top priorities of the day that will move the ball on your goals:

1. _____

2. _____

3. _____

## HYDRATION

Check off one droplet for each 8 ounces water you consume today.

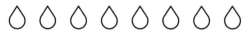

## MOVEMENT

What have I done today to move my body?

TRACKING CHARTS

295

## MEALS

**BREAKFAST:** _____

- ☐ Protein: _____
- ☐ Fat: _____
- ☐ Fiber: _____
- ☐ Greens: _____

**LUNCH:** _____

- ☐ Protein: _____
- ☐ Fat: _____
- ☐ Fiber: _____
- ☐ Greens: _____

**DINNER:** _____

- ☐ Protein: _____
- ☐ Fat: _____
- ☐ Fiber: _____
- ☐ Greens: _____

## POSITIVITY TRACKING

Write down three new and specific things you are grateful for today:

1.

2.

3.

## PARKING LOT

Write your thoughts and emotions out of your head and body and onto the page. Let go.

# Daily Expression

## Week 10/Date: _____

### HIT LIST

Write down three top priorities of the day that will move
the ball on your goals:

1. _____

2. _____

3. _____

### HYDRATION

Check off one droplet for each 8 ounces water you
consume today.

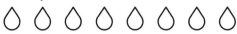

### MOVEMENT

What have I done today to move my body?

## MEALS

**BREAKFAST:** _____

- ☐ Protein: _____
- ☐ Fat: _____
- ☐ Fiber: _____
- ☐ Greens: _____


**LUNCH:** _____

- ☐ Protein: _____
- ☐ Fat: _____
- ☐ Fiber: _____
- ☐ Greens: _____


**DINNER:** _____

- ☐ Protein: _____
- ☐ Fat: _____
- ☐ Fiber: _____
- ☐ Greens: _____

## POSITIVITY TRACKING

Write down three new and specific things you are grateful for today:

*1.*

*2.*

*3.*

## PARKING LOT

Write your thoughts and emotions out of your head and body and onto the page. Let go.

# Daily Expression

**Week 10/Date: _____**

### HIT LIST

Write down three top priorities of the day that will move the ball on your goals:

*1.* _____

*2.* _____

*3.* _____

### HYDRATION

Check off one droplet for each 8 ounces water you consume today.

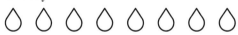

### MOVEMENT

What have I done today to move my body?

## MEALS

**BREAKFAST:** _____

☐ Protein: _____

☐ Fat: _____

☐ Fiber: _____

☐ Greens: _____


**LUNCH:** _____

☐ Protein: _____

☐ Fat: _____

☐ Fiber: _____

☐ Greens: _____


**DINNER:** _____

☐ Protein: _____

☐ Fat: _____

☐ Fiber: _____

☐ Greens: _____

## POSITIVITY TRACKING

Write down three new and specific things you are grateful for today:

1.

2.

3.

## PARKING LOT

Write your thoughts and emotions out of your head and body and onto the page. Let go.

# Daily Expression

**Week 10/Date:** _____

---

### HIT LIST

Write down three top priorities of the day that will move the ball on your goals:

1. _____

2. _____

3. _____

---

### HYDRATION

Check off one droplet for each 8 ounces water you consume today.

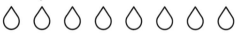

---

### MOVEMENT

What have I done today to move my body?

## MEALS

**BREAKFAST:** _____

☐  Protein: _____

☐  Fat: _____

☐  Fiber: _____

☐  Greens: _____


**LUNCH:** _____

☐  Protein: _____

☐  Fat: _____

☐  Fiber: _____

☐  Greens: _____


**DINNER:** _____

☐  Protein: _____

☐  Fat: _____

☐  Fiber: _____

☐  Greens: _____

## POSITIVITY TRACKING

Write down three new and specific things you are grateful for today:

1.

2.

3.

## PARKING LOT

Write your thoughts and emotions out of your head and body and onto the page. Let go.

# Daily Expression

**Week 10/Date: _____**

## HIT LIST

Write down three top priorities of the day that will move
the ball on your goals:

*1.* _____

*2.* _____

*3.* _____

## HYDRATION

Check off one droplet for each 8 ounces water you
consume today.

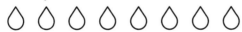

## MOVEMENT

What have I done today to move my body?

## MEALS

**BREAKFAST:** _____

☐ Protein: _____

☐ Fat: _____

☐ Fiber: _____

☐ Greens: _____


**LUNCH:** _____

☐ Protein: _____

☐ Fat: _____

☐ Fiber: _____

☐ Greens: _____


**DINNER:** _____

☐ Protein: _____

☐ Fat: _____

☐ Fiber: _____

☐ Greens: _____

## POSITIVITY TRACKING

Write down three new and specific things you are grateful for today:

*1.*

*2.*

.

*3.*

## PARKING LOT

Write your thoughts and emotions out of your head and body and onto the page. Let go.

# Daily Expression

**Week 10/Date: _____**

## HIT LIST

Write down three top priorities of the day that will move the ball on your goals:

1. _____

2. _____

3. _____

## HYDRATION

Check off one droplet for each 8 ounces water you consume today.

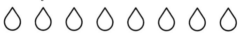

## MOVEMENT

What have I done today to move my body?

# MEALS

**BREAKFAST:** _____

☐ Protein: _____

☐ Fat: _____

☐ Fiber: _____

☐ Greens: _____


**LUNCH:** _____

☐ Protein: _____

☐ Fat: _____

☐ Fiber: _____

☐ Greens: _____


**DINNER:** _____

☐ Protein: _____

☐ Fat: _____

☐ Fiber: _____

☐ Greens: _____

## POSITIVITY TRACKING

Write down three new and specific things you are grateful for today:

1.

2.

3.

## PARKING LOT

Write your thoughts and emotions out of your head and body and onto the page. Let go.

# Weekly Planning

**Week 11:** _____

## SMOOTHIE INSPO

Write down three fun smoothie ideas for the next week:

1. _____

2. _____

3. _____

## #FAB4SMOOTHIE GROCERY LIST

☐ Liquid _____

   ☐   Nut Milk _____

   ☐   _____

☐ Protein _____

   ☐   Vanilla _____

   ☐   Chocolate _____

   ☐   _____

☐ Fat _____

   ☐   Avocado _____

   ☐   Nut Butter _____

   ☐   Coconut _____

   ☐   Healthy Oils _____

   ☐   _____

☐ Fiber _____

   ☐   Chia _____

   ☐   Flax _____

   ☐   Fiber Powders (acacia, psyllium husk)

☐ Greens _____

   ☐   Fresh _____

   ☐   Frozen _____

☐ Fruit _____

   ☐   Fresh _____

       ☐   Berries _____

       ☐   Citrus _____

       ☐   Tropical _____

   ☐   Frozen _____

       ☐   Berries _____

## WEEKLY MEAL PREP

Write down three great meal ideas for the next week:

1. _____

2. _____

3. _____

Which bulk protein do you want to use for your lunches?

_____

## FAB FOUR GROCERY LIST

☐ Protein

   ☐ _____

   ☐ _____

   ☐ _____

☐ Fat

   ☐ Cooking Oils _____

   ☐ Dressing _____

   ☐ Dip _____

☐ Nonstarchy Fiber-Rich Vegetables

☐ _____

☐ _____

☐ _____

☐ _____

☐ Greens

☐ Salad Greens _____

☐ Herbs _____

☐ Starch (one per week of savory and sweet)

☐ Savory _____

☐ Sweet _____

## ANCHOR APPOINTMENTS

**MONDAY**

**TUESDAY**

**WEDNESDAY**

**THURSDAY**

**FRIDAY**

**SATURDAY**

**SUNDAY**

# Daily Expression

## HIT LIST

Write down three top priorities of the day that will move the ball on your goals:

1. _____

2. _____

3. _____

## HYDRATION

Check off one droplet for each 8 ounces water you consume today.

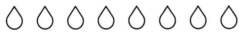

## MOVEMENT

What have I done today to move my body?

## MEALS

**BREAKFAST:** _____

☐ Protein: _____

☐ Fat: _____

☐ Fiber: _____

☐ Greens: _____


**LUNCH:** _____

☐ Protein: _____

☐ Fat: _____

☐ Fiber: _____

☐ Greens: _____


**DINNER:** _____

☐ Protein: _____

☐ Fat: _____

☐ Fiber: _____

☐ Greens: _____

## POSITIVITY TRACKING

Write down three new and specific things you are grateful for today:

1.

2.

3.

## PARKING LOT

Write your thoughts and emotions out of your head and body and onto the page. Let go.

# Daily Expression

## Week 11/Date: _____

### HIT LIST

Write down three top priorities of the day that will move the ball on your goals:

*1.* _____

*2.* _____

*3.* _____

### HYDRATION

Check off one droplet for each 8 ounces water you consume today.

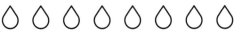

### MOVEMENT

What have I done today to move my body?

## MEALS

**BREAKFAST:** _____

☐ Protein: _____

☐ Fat: _____

☐ Fiber: _____

☐ Greens: _____


**LUNCH:** _____

☐ Protein: _____

☐ Fat: _____

☐ Fiber: _____

☐ Greens: _____


**DINNER:** _____

☐ Protein: _____

☐ Fat: _____

☐ Fiber: _____

☐ Greens: _____

TRACKING CHARTS

## POSITIVITY TRACKING

Write down three new and specific things you are grateful for today:

*1.*

*2.*

*3.*

## PARKING LOT

Write your thoughts and emotions out of your head and body and onto the page. Let go.

# Daily Expression

**Week 11/Date:** _____

---

**HIT LIST**

Write down three top priorities of the day that will move the ball on your goals:

1. _____

2. _____

3. _____

---

**HYDRATION**

Check off one droplet for each 8 ounces water you consume today.

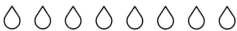

---

**MOVEMENT**

What have I done today to move my body?

## MEALS

**BREAKFAST:** _____

- ☐ Protein: _____
- ☐ Fat: _____
- ☐ Fiber: _____
- ☐ Greens: _____

**LUNCH:** _____

- ☐ Protein: _____
- ☐ Fat: _____
- ☐ Fiber: _____
- ☐ Greens: _____

**DINNER:** _____

- ☐ Protein: _____
- ☐ Fat: _____
- ☐ Fiber: _____
- ☐ Greens: _____

BODY LOVE A JOURNAL

## POSITIVITY TRACKING

Write down three new and specific things you are grateful for today:

*1.*

*2.*

*3.*

## PARKING LOT

Write your thoughts and emotions out of your head and body and onto the page. Let go.

# Daily Expression

**Week 11/Date:** _____

## HIT LIST

Write down three top priorities of the day that will move the ball on your goals:

*1.* _____

*2.* _____

*3.* _____

## HYDRATION

Check off one droplet for each 8 ounces water you consume today.

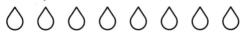

## MOVEMENT

What have I done today to move my body?

## MEALS

**BREAKFAST:** _____

☐ Protein: _____

☐ Fat: _____

☐ Fiber: _____

☐ Greens: _____


**LUNCH:** _____

☐ Protein: _____

☐ Fat: _____

☐ Fiber: _____

☐ Greens: _____


**DINNER:** _____

☐ Protein: _____

☐ Fat: _____

☐ Fiber: _____

☐ Greens: _____

## POSITIVITY TRACKING

Write down three new and specific things you are grateful for today:

1.

2.

3.

## PARKING LOT

Write your thoughts and emotions out of your head and body and onto the page. Let go.

# Daily Expression

**Week 11/Date:** _____

## HIT LIST

Write down three top priorities of the day that will move the ball on your goals:

*1.* _____

*2.* _____

*3.* _____

## HYDRATION

Check off one droplet for each 8 ounces water you consume today.

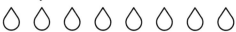

## MOVEMENT

What have I done today to move my body?

**BREAKFAST:** _____

☐ Protein: _____

☐ Fat: _____

☐ Fiber: _____

☐ Greens: _____


**LUNCH:** _____

☐ Protein: _____

☐ Fat: _____

☐ Fiber: _____

☐ Greens: _____


**DINNER:** _____

☐ Protein: _____

☐ Fat: _____

☐ Fiber: _____

☐ Greens: _____

BODY LOVE A JOURNAL

## POSITIVITY TRACKING

Write down three new and specific things you are grateful for today:

1.

2.

3.

## PARKING LOT

Write your thoughts and emotions out of your head and body and onto the page. Let go.

# Daily Expression

**Week 11/Date:** _____

## HIT LIST

Write down three top priorities of the day that will move the ball on your goals:

1. _____

2. _____

3. _____

## HYDRATION

Check off one droplet for each 8 ounces water you consume today.

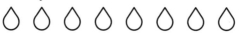

## MOVEMENT

What have I done today to move my body?

## MEALS

**BREAKFAST:** _____

☐ Protein: _____

☐ Fat: _____

☐ Fiber: _____

☐ Greens: _____


**LUNCH:** _____

☐ Protein: _____

☐ Fat: _____

☐ Fiber: _____

☐ Greens: _____


**DINNER:** _____

☐ Protein: _____

☐ Fat: _____

☐ Fiber: _____

☐ Greens: _____

## POSITIVITY TRACKING

Write down three new and specific things you are grateful for today:

*1.*

*2.*

*3.*

## PARKING LOT

Write your thoughts and emotions out of your head and body and onto the page. Let go.

# Daily Expression

## HIT LIST

Write down three top priorities of the day that will move the ball on your goals:

*1.* _____

*2.* _____

*3.* _____

## HYDRATION

Check off one droplet for each 8 ounces water you consume today.

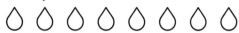

## MOVEMENT

What have I done today to move my body?

## MEALS

**BREAKFAST:** _____

- ☐ Protein: _____
- ☐ Fat: _____
- ☐ Fiber: _____
- ☐ Greens: _____


**LUNCH:** _____

- ☐ Protein: _____
- ☐ Fat: _____
- ☐ Fiber: _____
- ☐ Greens: _____


**DINNER:** _____

- ☐ Protein: _____
- ☐ Fat: _____
- ☐ Fiber: _____
- ☐ Greens: _____

## POSITIVITY TRACKING

Write down three new and specific things you are grateful for today:

*1.*

*2.*

*3.*

## PARKING LOT

Write your thoughts and emotions out of your head and body and onto the page. Let go.

# Weekly Planning

## SMOOTHIE INSPO

Write down three fun smoothie ideas for the next week:

*1.* _____

*2.* _____

*3.* _____

## #FAB4SMOOTHIE GROCERY LIST

☐ Liquid _____

   ☐    Nut Milk _____

   ☐    _____

☐ Protein _____

   ☐    Vanilla _____

   ☐    Chocolate _____

   ☐    _____

- ☐ Fat _____
  - ☐    Avocado _____
  - ☐    Nut Butter _____
  - ☐    Coconut _____
  - ☐    Healthy Oils _____
  - ☐    _____
- ☐ Fiber _____
  - ☐    Chia _____
  - ☐    Flax _____
  - ☐    Fiber Powders (acacia, psyllium husk) _____
- ☐ Greens _____
  - ☐    Fresh _____
  - ☐    Frozen _____
- ☐ Fruit _____
  - ☐    Fresh _____
    - ☐    Berries _____
    - ☐    Citrus _____
    - ☐    Tropical _____
  - ☐    Frozen _____
    - ☐    Berries _____

Write down three great meal ideas for the next week:

*1.* _____

*2.* _____

*3.* _____

Which bulk protein do you want to use for your lunches?

_____

## FAB FOUR GROCERY LIST

- ☐ Protein
  - ☐ _____
  - ☐ _____
  - ☐ _____

- ☐ Fat
  - ☐ Cooking Oils _____
  - ☐ Dressing _____
  - ☐ Dip _____

- ☐ Nonstarchy Fiber-Rich Vegetables

  - ☐ _____

  - ☐ _____

  - ☐ _____

  - ☐ _____

- ☐ Greens

  - ☐ Salad Greens _____

  - ☐ Herbs _____

- ☐ Starch (one per week of savory and sweet)

  - ☐ Savory _____

  - ☐ Sweet _____

## ANCHOR APPOINTMENTS

**MONDAY**

**TUESDAY**

**WEDNESDAY**

**THURSDAY**

**FRIDAY**

**SATURDAY**

**SUNDAY**

# Daily Expression

**Week 12/Date:** _____

## HIT LIST

Write down three top priorities of the day that will move
the ball on your goals:

*1.* _____

*2.* _____

*3.* _____

## HYDRATION

Check off one droplet for each 8 ounces water you
consume today.

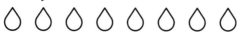

## MOVEMENT

What have I done today to move my body?

# MEALS

**BREAKFAST:** _____

☐ Protein: _____

☐ Fat: _____

☐ Fiber: _____

☐ Greens: _____


**LUNCH:** _____

☐ Protein: _____

☐ Fat: _____

☐ Fiber: _____

☐ Greens: _____


**DINNER:** _____

☐ Protein: _____

☐ Fat: _____

☐ Fiber: _____

☐ Greens: _____

TRACKING CHARTS

## POSITIVITY TRACKING

Write down three new and specific things you are grateful for today:

1.

2.

3.

## PARKING LOT

Write your thoughts and emotions out of your head and body and onto the page. Let go.

# Daily Expression

**Week 12/Date:** _____

### HIT LIST

Write down three top priorities of the day that will move the ball on your goals:

1. _____

2. _____

3. _____

### HYDRATION

Check off one droplet for each 8 ounces water you consume today.

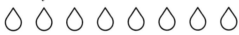

### MOVEMENT

What have I done today to move my body?

345

**BREAKFAST:** _____

☐ Protein: _____

☐ Fat: _____

☐ Fiber: _____

☐ Greens: _____


**LUNCH:** _____

☐ Protein: _____

☐ Fat: _____

☐ Fiber: _____

☐ Greens: _____


**DINNER:** _____

☐ Protein: _____

☐ Fat: _____

☐ Fiber: _____

☐ Greens: _____

BODY LOVE A JOURNAL

## POSITIVITY TRACKING

Write down three new and specific things you are grateful for today:

1.

2.

3.

## PARKING LOT

Write your thoughts and emotions out of your head and body and onto the page. Let go.

# Daily Expression

**Week 12/Date:** _____

## HIT LIST

Write down three top priorities of the day that will move the ball on your goals:

1. _____

2. _____

3. _____

## HYDRATION

Check off one droplet for each 8 ounces water you consume today.

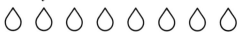

## MOVEMENT

What have I done today to move my body?

## MEALS

**BREAKFAST:** _____

- ☐ Protein: _____
- ☐ Fat: _____
- ☐ Fiber: _____
- ☐ Greens: _____

**LUNCH:** _____

- ☐ Protein: _____
- ☐ Fat: _____
- ☐ Fiber: _____
- ☐ Greens: _____

**DINNER:** _____

- ☐ Protein: _____
- ☐ Fat: _____
- ☐ Fiber: _____
- ☐ Greens: _____

TRACKING CHARTS

## POSITIVITY TRACKING

Write down three new and specific things you are grateful for today:

1.

2.

3.

## PARKING LOT

Write your thoughts and emotions out of your head and body and onto the page. Let go.

# Daily Expression

## HIT LIST

Write down three top priorities of the day that will move
the ball on your goals:

1. _____

2. _____

3. _____

## HYDRATION

Check off one droplet for each 8 ounces water you
consume today.

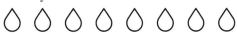

## MOVEMENT

What have I done today to move my body?

TRACKING CHARTS

## MEALS

**BREAKFAST:** _____

☐ Protein: _____

☐ Fat: _____

☐ Fiber: _____

☐ Greens: _____


**LUNCH:** _____

☐ Protein: _____

☐ Fat: _____

☐ Fiber: _____

☐ Greens: _____


**DINNER:** _____

☐ Protein: _____

☐ Fat: _____

☐ Fiber: _____

☐ Greens: _____

## POSITIVITY TRACKING

Write down three new and specific things you are grateful for today:

1.

2.

3.

## PARKING LOT

Write your thoughts and emotions out of your head and body and onto the page. Let go.

# Daily Expression

## Week 12/Date: _____

### HIT LIST

Write down three top priorities of the day that will move the ball on your goals:

1. _____

2. _____

3. _____

### HYDRATION

Check off one droplet for each 8 ounces water you consume today.

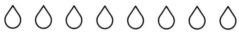

### MOVEMENT

What have I done today to move my body?

## MEALS

**BREAKFAST:** _____

☐ Protein: _____

☐ Fat: _____

☐ Fiber: _____

☐ Greens: _____


**LUNCH:** _____

☐ Protein: _____

☐ Fat: _____

☐ Fiber: _____

☐ Greens: _____


**DINNER:** _____

☐ Protein: _____

☐ Fat: _____

☐ Fiber: _____

☐ Greens: _____

## POSITIVITY TRACKING

Write down three new and specific things you are grateful for today:

*1.*

*2.*

*3.*

## PARKING LOT

Write your thoughts and emotions out of your head and body and onto the page. Let go.

# Daily Expression

**Week 12/Date:** _____

### HIT LIST

Write down three top priorities of the day that will move the ball on your goals:

1. _____

2. _____

3. _____

### HYDRATION

Check off one droplet for each 8 ounces water you consume today.

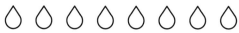

### MOVEMENT

What have I done today to move my body?

## MEALS

**BREAKFAST:** _____

☐ Protein: _____

☐ Fat: _____

☐ Fiber: _____

☐ Greens: _____


**LUNCH:** _____

☐ Protein: _____

☐ Fat: _____

☐ Fiber: _____

☐ Greens: _____


**DINNER:** _____

☐ Protein: _____

☐ Fat: _____

☐ Fiber: _____

☐ Greens: _____

## POSITIVITY TRACKING

Write down three new and specific things you are grateful for today:

*1.*

*2.*

*3.*

## PARKING LOT

Write your thoughts and emotions out of your head and body and onto the page. Let go.

# Daily Expression

**Week 12/Date:** _____

### HIT LIST

Write down three top priorities of the day that will move the ball on your goals:

1. _____

2. _____

3. _____

### HYDRATION

Check off one droplet for each 8 ounces water you consume today.

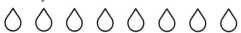

### MOVEMENT

What have I done today to move my body?

# MEALS

**BREAKFAST:** _____

☐ Protein: _____

☐ Fat: _____

☐ Fiber: _____

☐ Greens: _____


**LUNCH:** _____

☐ Protein: _____

☐ Fat: _____

☐ Fiber: _____

☐ Greens: _____


**DINNER:** _____

☐ Protein: _____

☐ Fat: _____

☐ Fiber: _____

☐ Greens: _____

TRACKING CHARTS

## POSITIVITY TRACKING

Write down three new and specific things you are grateful
for today:

*1.*

*2.*

*3.*

## PARKING LOT

Write your thoughts and emotions out of your head and
body and onto the page. Let go.

# Monthly Manifestation

**Month:** _____

## GO IN

Identify self-limiting beliefs and emotional patterns
holding you back.

## LET GO

Take a moment to forgive yourself, release resentment,
and erase regrets. It's time to let go of these beliefs and
move forward.

## MANIFEST MAGIC

With nothing holding you back, visualize what your life would look like in a month, a year, five years, and ten years from now and write it down, being as specific as possible.

## MONTHLY SMART GOALS

Using the SMART goals framework on page 41, be specific about the repeatable and actionable steps you plan to take this month.

1. _____

2. _____

3. _____

# REFLECTIONS

Using the prompts below, reflect on your experience with Body Love?

1. What have you learned about yourself through this practice?

_____

_____

_____

_____

_____

_____

2. How has your relationship with food changed in the last three months?

_____

_____

_____

_____

_____

_____

3. What practices have enriched your life most? How do you plan to carry that technique forward in your life?

_____

_____

_____

_____

_____

_____

# ABOUT KELLY LEVEQUE AND BODY LOVE

**KELLY LeVEQUE** is a holistic nutritionist, wellness expert, celebrity health coach, and the bestselling author of *Body Love* and *Body Love Every Day.* Her deep desire to help her clients, her passion for human nutrition, and her curiosity about how and why the body works drive Kelly to diligently study the latest research, evaluate competing theories, and use this information to make individualized recommendations for her clients. Most important, Kelly's practical and always optimistic approach to nutrition and

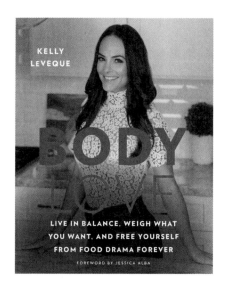

KELLY LeVEQUE

**BODY LOVE**

LIVE IN BALANCE, WEIGH WHAT YOU WANT, AND FREE YOURSELF FROM FOOD DRAMA FOREVER

FOREWORD BY JESSICA ALBA

wellness helps her readers improve their health, achieve their goals, and develop sustainable habits to live healthy and balanced lives.

Kelly's website serves as a resource for her readers to find the latest research and rationales behind important nutritional principles, as well as delicious recipes and recommended products to fuel them well. In 2020, she launched the *Be Well by Kelly* podcast to further provide listeners with her nutrition and wellness wisdom and to introduce them to other health professionals with a wide array of experience and insights. With the desire to provide her coaching expertise to the public, Kelly developed the Fab Four Fundamentals course, in which she simplifies the science of nutrition and empowers participants to confidently take charge of their health. Additionally, Kelly released the Be Well by Kelly LeVeque Protein Powder to round out the Body Love toolkit. This protein powder harnesses the power and benefits of simple yet wholesome protein and can easily be used in one of Kelly's favorite tools, the #fab4smoothie. Through all these resources, Kelly seeks to provide women with the tools they need to transform their health and their lives through nourishing whole foods and body-loving practices.

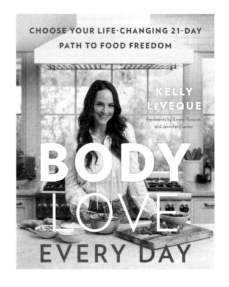

Kelly created this journal for you to live the body-loving practices she uses with her clients, and she wants to hear from you! Tag your Body Love journal experience with the hashtag #BodyLoveJournal!